The *Source*
for
Dyslexia
and
Dysgraphia

Regina G. Richards

Skill Areas:	Dyslexia and Dysgraphia
Age Level:	All ages

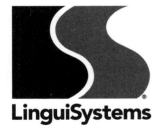

LinguiSystems

LinguiSystems, Inc.
3100 4th Avenue
East Moline, IL 61244

800-776-4332

FAX: 800-577-4555
E-mail: service@linguisystems.com
Web: linguisystems.com

Printed in the U.S.A.

ISBN 10: 0-7606-0308-1
ISBN 13: 978-0-7606-0308-6

About the Author

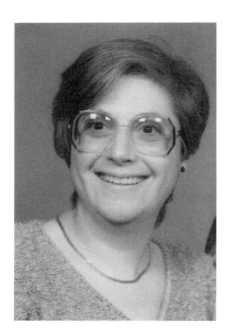

Regina G. Richards, M.A. is a Director of Richards Educational Therapy Center and Big Springs School, which specializes in multidisciplinary programs for language learning disabilities, especially dyslexia and dysgraphia. As an educational therapist, she has been practicing in Riverside, California, since 1975. She began her career in bilingual education, working on curriculum development and test design, and has authored a variety of journal articles and books on visual development, reading, dyslexia, and dysgraphia. She was president of the Inland Empire Branch of the International Dyslexia Association for seven years and has been editor of the annual IDA California Cosortium's Resource Directory since 1992. Since 1970, she has presented workshops and classes at the University of California Extension Programs at both the Riverside and San Diego campuses and she speaks at conferences and workshops nationally. *The Source for Dyslexia and Dysgraphia* is Regina's first publication with LinguiSystems.

Acknowledgements

Ideas, ideas, ideas . . . where have my ideas come from? . . . books, colleagues, conference speakers, networking at conferences, teachers taking my classes, the list goes on and on. It's impossible to evaluate the depth of the influence others have had on the development of my philosophies. But I give my sincere thanks to each and every one of you. I am especially indebted to the wonderful and talented staff at the Richards Educational Therapy Center and Big Springs School for the many discussions about students, philosophies, techniques, strategies, developmental sequences, etc. Thank you to the speech and language pathologists, Andrea Newall and Dindy Wheelock; and to the educational therapists, Simone Acosta, Jeff Bleszinski, Judy Love, Pam Meeker, Betty Meeks, JoAnn Morris, and Sally Smith. Thanks also to Julie Greenwalt, assistant office manager at RETC, for the numerous hours of typing required by a project as involved as this. Also, thanks to Steven Kerekes, special education resource specialist, and Alan Kwasman, M.D., pediatrician, for their comments and for previewing parts of the manuscript. Special thanks to Melvin D. Levine, M.D. and Martha S. Reed, M.Ed., from the Center for the Development and Learning at the University of North Carolina, Chapel Hill, for the wonderful and inspirational six-day class I took in August 1995. I learned so much from these talented people—especially how to look at students with a phenomenological approach, rather than a pure labeling approach.

I thank the countless students I've worked with over the years, and perhaps these fine youngsters have had the greatest influence on my philosophies. Their frustrations, stamina, and most especially, their courage, have motivated me to continue to seek for alternative and more specific techniques and strategies.

A special thank you goes to Eli. Thank you, Eli, for being Eli and for all of your sharing. Thank you also to my wonderful husband, Irv, for his continual support and endless patience and encouragement.

This book is dedicated to
Dovid M. Richards,
forever in my heart

Table of Contents

Table of Contents

There is a very long history of development behind this book, even though the phase from outline to printing was only slightly more than a year.

The seeds of this project germinated in 1983 as a result of my frustration in trying to describe my son to his preschool teachers. At that point I had been an educational professional within the community for about a decade. I was running a school and clinic, and I was very active in the International Dyslexia Association. I knew my young son and I understood why he seemed to be "two different kids" to his teachers. The kid they saw during playtime and storytime was very different from the kid they observed during writing and alphabet time.

I experienced a conundrum. Using a label to describe my son led to a great deal of misunderstanding, as every teacher had her own definition for whatever word I chose to use. Describing my son was useful, but time-consuming. For a while I used the phrase "he learns differently," but this was not sufficient as he progressed in elementary school. After all, he could read, but there was a qualitative difference in how he approached and processed language-based tasks. At that point I developed the philosophy that "a label without a description is useless, but a description without a label is not always efficient."

I would describe my son to his teachers, then identify a classification, saying, "These are the characteristics of his *dyslexia* (and later *dysgraphia*) that affect his performances in the classroom" or "This is how his *attention* is affected by the language load of the lesson." It seemed to me that this approach facilitated communication. People like to have a handle, a shortcut, and a reference point. But I needed to be sure that they understood which of my son's characteristics affected his learning, and how the interaction between the characteristics worked.

The philosophy, "a label without a description is useless, but a description without a label is not always efficient," has stayed with me throughout my professional career and has been very useful in my university teaching, my remedial work with students, and especially in explaining students to their parents after an evaluation. I hope that you will consider adapting this philosophy in dealing with your students. Please help avoid the pigeonholing and empty labeling that comes with the mere use of a label. Those practices can be so damaging to students. Be sure to always describe your student, ideally by looking for commonalities among his characteristics, so that you can discuss the patterns that apply. Once everyone is aware of the description, then you can use the label, if it meets your needs for additional communication.

Many of my publications have started out with a desire to share information about my son and how he learns in an effort to help him and other students like him. I used the materials from my practice because I knew from my clinical experience that these methods worked. I initially wrote *LEARN: playful techniques to accelerate learning* in 1993 as a compilation of multisensory learning strategies. That book is now out of print and many of the tried-and-true strategies are incorporated in this new publication. In 1995, after several years of research and exploration, I wrote the pamphlet, *When writing's a problem,* to help parents and teachers understand the group of bright students who struggle to produce neat papers. I think this may be among the most misunderstood group of students in our educational system today. Because of multiple requests to expand this pamphlet to include a variety of teaching and remedial strategies, I then wrote *The Writing Dilemma: understanding dysgraphia* in 1998. *The Source for Dyslexia and Dysgraphia* is an expansion of *The Writing Dilemma* and incorporates many of its ideas and strategies. But these strategies are also integrated with a more extensive discussion of and strategies for the basic reading and spelling processes.

Dr. Melvin D. Levine, professor of pediatrics at the University of North Carolina Medical School; Director of the I; and Founding President of All Kinds of Minds, a nonprofit institute for the Understanding of Differences in Learning, wrote a wonderful foreword for *The Writing Dilemma.* His title was *What's Riding on Writing.* A few quotes are pertinent here:

> "Writing represents the ultimate neurocognitive integrative act. It is the supreme accomplishment of a developing young mind. It is in the act of writing and only in the act of writing that a seemingly diverse collection of germinating neurodevelopmental functions and academic subskills coalesce and collaborate. Writing demands the vigorous participation of attention, multiple forms of memory, language, critical and creative thought, brainstorming, motor output, megacognition, progressive automization, organization, synchronization, and even visualization. In addition, writing represents a formidable challenge to problem-solving skills, as exigencies, such as planning, previewing, topic selection, strategy use, self-monitoring, and pacing represent core components of the problem-solving act . . . .

> "There exist a multitude of possible reasons (and very common combinations of reasons) for a student's writing failure or reluctance. Consequently, there are as many subtypes of writing disorders. When we come to understand the reasons for a particular child's writing difficulty, we have learned an enormous amount about that individual's intrinsic 'writing' . . . .

> "Up until now, writing has been a well-guarded territory, narrowly divided between professional disciplines . . . Clearly, it is time for a holistic approach to the understanding of writing and of problems with writing. *The Writing Dilemma* offers to the educational world an embarrassingly overdue breakthrough, as this most important work acknowledges and describes vividly the multiple possible breakdown points that must be considered in a child who is not developing writing skills . . . .

> "No child needs or deserves to suffer writing humiliation, we assert penitently!"

Thank you, Dr. Levine, for putting the problem in such clear perspective. *The Source for Dyslexia and Dysgraphia* seeks to expand my holistic approach to the understanding of writing, integrating it with an understanding of reading. This book takes a thorough look at the areas of reading and writing, omitting comprehension because that opens another whole domain.

It is my hope and wish that the information and strategies included in this book are useful in helping you describe and understand the child or children within your sphere of concern, and that you and the children have fun in your work together. To expand on Dr. Levine's marvelous "Tom Swifty" (see chapter 13 for more):

> No child needs or deserves to suffer the embarrassment of being unable to read, I proclaim soundly!

Regina

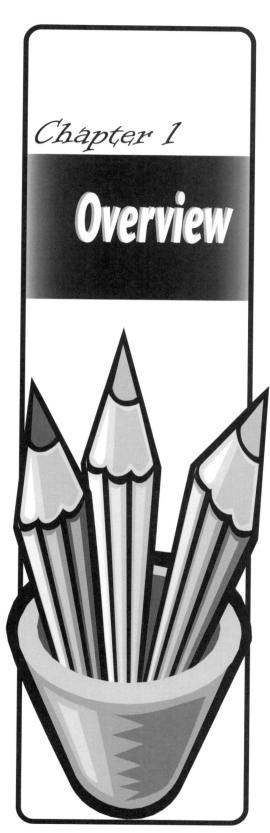

Chapter 1

Overview

As a toddler, Eli was very curious and enthusiastic. He loved to explore, stopping often to "smell the roses." These frequent distractions sometimes caused him to disappear in an instant. During the crawling stage, he would crawl under furniture to explore a speck of dust. As he began to walk more efficiently, his parents put bells on his shoes to keep track of him. Everything was new and exciting and of great interest to Eli, including unscrewing the bolts on the legs of his crib. His family visited their future house when Eli was a year old and he became lost. There was no furniture in the house, all the doors were closed, and he was not yet walking. His parents couldn't guess where he was hiding. Eventually they found him sitting in the fireplace (fortunately not in use), playing with the ashes. He had crawled behind the grate and became fascinated by the ashes and the slight breeze that was coming down the chimney.

Eli began babbling quite early and appeared to have a fast-developing vocabulary. As his vocabulary grew, it became evident that he had difficulty saying multi-syllabic words. Words with repeating or similar syllables were easy (*mama, dada*), but he sometimes reversed the syllables in a word such as *cookie* and said "keecoo." As he progressed to phrases, his sequencing problems continued. His favorite cartoon was "RunRoader" and he enjoyed playing with the "ball base-bat." He had a good ability to memorize nursery rhymes and communicate; however, many of the words he used were mixed up or he substituted syllables. He began to sing the alphabet (with his own style of substitutions) at around age three or four. As his preschool class began learning alphabet letters, he experienced tremendous difficulty and became good at avoiding such activities.

Everyone seemed to love Eli; he was very personable, extremely curious, and full of adventure. Because of his continuing difficulties with sequences of sounds in words and learning alphabet letters, he was placed in a private school that offered a sequential, well-organized, and precise phonics-based reading program. He also received after-school tutoring using the Orton-Gillingham method—a multisensory, structured, systematic phonics program. Eli seemed to be full of paradoxes. He appeared so bright, so curious, and highly mechanical. He was great at class discussions and demonstrated a ready grasp of complex concepts. However, he struggled greatly with reading and writing, even at a very young age.

By second grade, Eli was reading at grade level and he loved writing stories, especially when he was allowed to use his own creative spelling. However, as he progressed in school he wrote less and less. He explained, "Writing is not fun anymore. There are too many things to think about—periods, capital letters, and all that." He was very frustrated with the difficulty he experienced in trying to create a neat paper, and he constantly complained about the teacher's "mean comments about how sloppy I am." (Figure 1.1 on page 13 illustrates Eli's difficulty with the mechanics of writing.) No matter how hard he tried, it was a struggle to make his writing neat. When he worked hard and came close to being neat, it took him an extreme amount of time and he was very fatigued by the end of the first line. Fortunately for Eli, he picked up keyboarding at an early age and his teachers allowed him to type lengthy papers and assignments.

Eli reports that music and pictures are constantly flowing in his head. As a youngster the music would sometimes escape and he would sing out during class. As he matured, he learned to monitor his behavior and keep the song inside. He has also learned to control some of his tendencies to daydream. The constant internal background of music and visuals is part of the reason it is hard for him to maintain attention while reading, even as a college student. Despite these characteristics, many neurologists and neuropsychologists through the years have ruled out a diagnosis of Attention Deficit Disorder.

Eli is extremely skilled at visual cues, including reading people's moods and intentions (nonverbal awareness) and spatial awareness. He always remembers where he has been and where he is going, and seems to have a natural ability to find his way through the environment. He was frustrated as a youngster because he could find his way through a shopping mall and he knew exactly where a store was, but he could not read or remember the name of the store. He understands time concepts but has substantial difficulty reading an analog clock. Even as a college student, he sometimes counts by fives to figure out the correct time on an analog clock, or he has to stop and think whether *two forty-five* is the same as *quarter to three*.

Figure 1.1—*The Chick's Cracked Egg*, a story by Eli, written in third grade

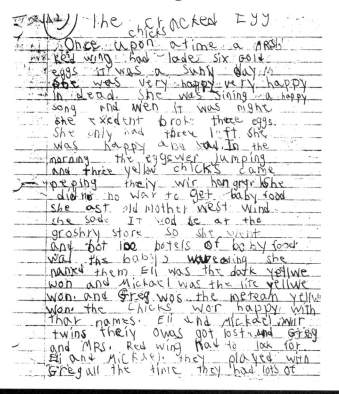

Translation of Eli's story (with corrected spelling):

Once upon a time, a Mrs. Red Wing had laid six gold eggs. It was a sunny day. She was very happy, very happy indeed. She was singing a happy song and when it was night she accidentally broke three eggs. She only had three left. She was happy and sad. In the morning, the eggs were jumping and three yellow chicks came peeping (out). They were hungry. She didn't know where to get baby food. She asked old Mother West Wind. She said it would be at the grocery store. So she went and bought 100 bottles of baby food. While the babies were eating she named them. Eli was the dark yellow one and Michael was the light yellow one. And Greg was the medium yellow one. The chicks were happy with their names. Eli and Michael were twins. They always got lost and Greg and Mrs. Red Wing had to look for Eli and Michael. They played with Greg all the time. They had lots of fun together. Greg ate a lot of food. He was fat. But Eli and Michael hated to eat. They were very skinny. You can see right through them and you can hardly see them. And one day Eli and Michael got fat. They ate more than Greg.

What's Going On?

Is Eli dyslexic? Yes. Is Eli dysgraphic? Yes. Both were diagnosed by a neuropsychologist when Eli was seven years old. Does either label matter? No, it is much more beneficial to describe Eli's strengths and weaknesses. Then why should we use the terms *dyslexia* and *dysgraphia*? Using either term provides a *shortcut* to help the listener relate Eli's profile to a generalized profile of someone who struggles with written language.

Eli demonstrated many high-risk symptoms as a preschooler:

- ✔ poor sound sequencing
- ✔ difficulty recalling words
- ✔ sound substitutions
- ✔ difficulty learning letters

As he entered school, his struggles with reading and writing became more pronounced. Fortunately, Eli was placed in appropriate programs and has learned beneficial skills. Even so, he still has great difficulty with the mechanics of reading and writing. He sometimes gets around his problems because of his astuteness at reading people and his ability to figure out some of his teachers. For example, as a high school senior he determined that his government teacher did not always read the quizzes; if he just wrote a substantial amount, he received credit for his efforts. In these example questions (Figure 1.2), he was given an A for a quiz that required him to answer 10 questions copied from the chalkboard.

Figure 1.2 — Eli's sample test answers

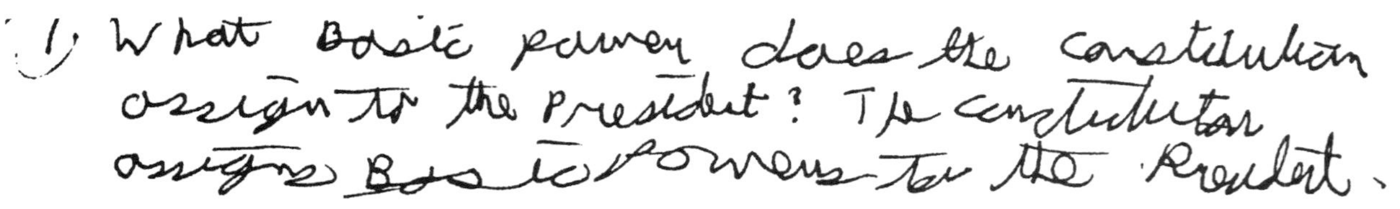

Translation: What basic power does the Constitution assign to the President? The Constitution assigns basic powers to the President.

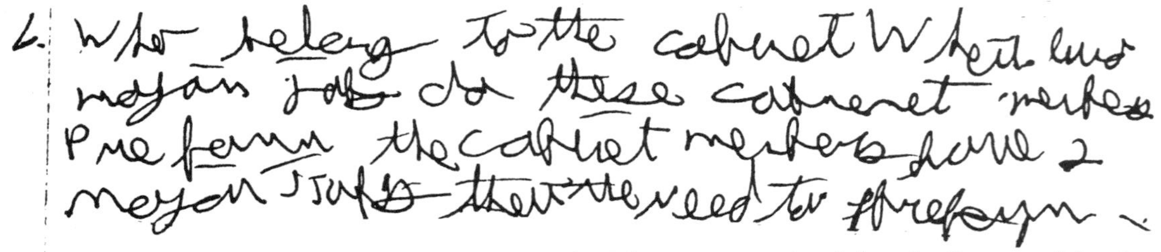

Translation: Who belongs to the cabinet? What two major jobs do these cabinet members perform? The cabinet members have two major jobs that the (they) need to perform.

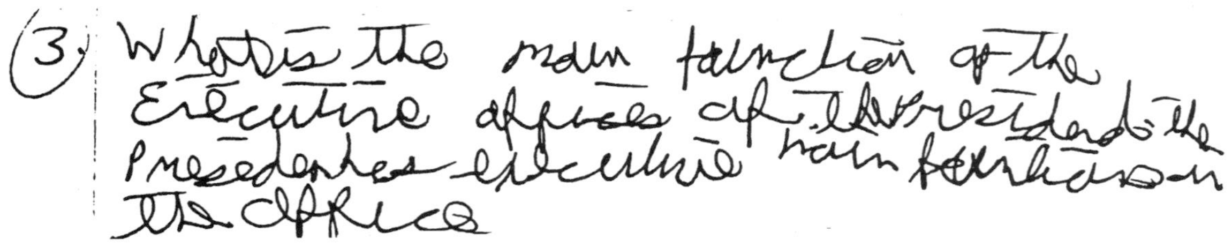

Translation: What is the main function of the executive offices of the President? The President's executive main function is the office.

While this strategy is not recommended as an enhancement of the learning process, it represents this student's way of coping with a large volume of work.

The key factors enabling Eli to function adequately within the educational system were helping him feel good about himself as a learner, feel confident talking to teachers, and develop self-advocacy skills. As he matured, he realized that his self-advocacy skills, which were based on self-understanding, led to his growth in confidence and ability to deal with a variety of educational situations.

Two days before he began high school, his special education case carrier called a meeting of all Eli's teachers. Each of his six teachers attended, along with the school psychologist, Eli, and his parents. The goal was to introduce and explain Eli to his teachers. At his parent's request, the words *dyslexia* and *dysgraphia* were never used. Rather, Eli's strengths and weaknesses were described, along with recommendations for accommodations.

Eli received much praise from his teachers for attending that meeting. They explained that few students bothered, although they were always invited. From that experience, Eli learned the value of introducing himself and explaining that he had many strengths, but also that certain tasks would cause him difficulty. At the beginning of each semester, he went to his new teachers, provided a copy of his IEP (Individual Education Plan), and explained his strengths and weaknesses. As he matured, his explanations became clearer—from his statements of only a few words to full sentences. Developing self-advocacy is a *process*, a critical one that greatly enhanced Eli's success levels.

Two Goals of This Book

For many children the risk signs for a significant struggle with reading and writing are not identified early. Such students unfortunately experience many years of frustration and lowered feelings of self-worth in the school environment, often resulting in wasted potential. When the risk signs are identified early, the student can be supported and helped through the educational process.

Goal #1: The first goal is to describe the processing styles inherent in dyslexia and dysgraphia in sufficient detail to allow you to identify such students with a degree of confidence. The goal is not necessarily to assign a label. What is important is to identify students who are at-risk because of processing problems that interfere with their ability to develop efficient reading and writing skills.

Hence, it is critical to only use a label with a corresponding description. The label helps the readers/listeners focus their understanding toward a specific category, but only the description can help them understand the child; the label aids communication, but only the more global aspects.

Is it a dream to want every student to feel comfortable and successful? No, it is not a dream. It can be achieved with a huge dose of understanding and a moderate dose of strategies. Dr. Mel Levine frequently states that the best *prescription* begins with a thorough *description*. (Levine 1998)

Goal #2: The second goal of this book is to describe strategies and compensations for students who struggle with academic skills. These strategies are useful for any student who would benefit by increased efficiency and automaticity. Because dyslexic and dysgraphic students are often disorganized in how they learn, organized and systematic instruction will benefit them because they are more likely to grasp and retain that information. Consequently, these strategies, while useful for many, may be *essential* for dyslexic or dysgraphic students.

Part Two of this book (beginning on page 91) begins with a discussion of the decision to either compensate or remediate and ends with direct strategy suggestions to enhance recall. The subsequent chapters describe remedial techniques for reading, spelling, and writing. These techniques don't represent a full literacy development program, as many extensive programs are on the market. Rather, the reading, spelling, and writing strategies are designed to supplement an existing language arts program by providing techniques that are particularly beneficial for the dyslexic or dysgraphic student. They can be used with students of any age who need assistance at that developmental level. The area of reading comprehension has been omitted because students with dyslexic processing problems benefit from almost any well-sequenced comprehension program that provides direct teaching, rather than merely multiple opportunities for practice.

Why Combine Dyslexia and Dysgraphia?

The strategies for dyslexia and dysgraphia are combined in this book because both of these processing differences are language-based and represent a struggle with written language. In reading, the struggle is basically receiving, or interpreting, the written language. The processing base of dyslexia involves poor integration of language components. For some, it may be an ability to grasp and manipulate sound units whereas for others it may have more effect on units of meaning. The processing base for dysgraphia involves poor motor planning, which affects the retrieval or production of written language.

The following list of similarities between these two processing styles reveals why many students may experience both struggles.

Similarities Between Dyslexia and Dysgraphia

- Both have a poor processing base causing sequencing struggles: poor ability to organize information or movements in a specific automatic order

- Both involve a struggle to develop automaticity of overall performances: skill performance is labored, resulting in decreased efficiency and poor automatic use

- Both involve a struggle with automatic visual recognition and/or retrieval of letter form

- Both benefit from similar strategies:
  - ✔ Systematic instruction
  - ✔ Multisensory techniques
  - ✔ Focus on making connections
  - ✔ Staging (performing one subtask at a time)

- Both benefit from similar compensations:
  - ✔ External assistance (books on tape or dictation of papers)
  - ✔ Extra time

The overall intent of this book is to help you better understand the struggles experienced by dyslexic and dysgraphic students, as well as appreciate the amazing gifts exhibited by these students. Many times such students appear to be paradoxes. What is typically easy for others (such as reading small words or performing elementary math tasks) may actually be very difficult for dyslexic students. Conversely, what is hard for others provides areas for the dyslexic students to shine, primarily because of their brightness and creativity. Eileen Simpson, a dyslexic, struggled with rote, mechanical knowledge. However, she began to excel in high school when she was allowed to take courses such as logic and philosophy because her ability to deal with abstractions was highly developed. (Simpson 1979, 153) As teachers and parents, we need to focus on helping all students find their way to shine in the academic world.

Some adult dyslexics who are gifted musicians and songwriters have expressed these same ideas in a poetic manner. Here's an example in song form by Josie Burns, a musician and artist.

The Select Few 🎵   Words and Music by Josie Burns

There are many of us out there,
Who march to a different beat,
Like Einstein and da Vinci,
Folks you'd really like to meet.

In music & art & science,
We're prone to excel,
But in your classrooms,
We're more than likely to fail.

(Chorus)
So give us a hug,
And hold tightly to our hand,
We'll take you exploring,
Into our wonderland.

You wanted us to be perfect,
When we were just brand new,
You wanted us to "fit in,"
When we're among a select few.

So then you called us "lazy,"
And said we could if we tried;
Why don't you try to see us,
Through . . . God's eyes.

(Chorus)
So give us a hug,
And hold tightly to our hand,
We'll take you exploring,
Into our wonderland.

You'll find there's very little,
That we cannot do,
And maybe you'll find out,
We can, even better than you.

(Chorus)
So give us a hug,
And hold tightly to our hand,
We'll take you exploring,
Into our wonderland.

Copyright © 1988, Josie Burns
Used with permission.

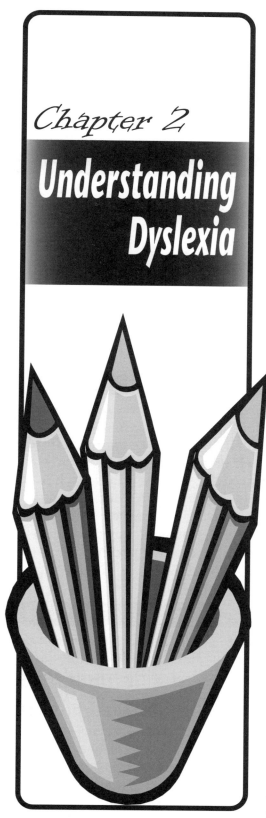

Chapter 2

Understanding Dyslexia

Dyslexia is one of the **learning** differences that has been greatly misunderstood throughout educational history. These misunderstandings have resulted in many myths that have been disproven by analysis, experience, and/or research. We need to ask why there are so many myths surrounding this learning pattern. A contributing factor is that dyslexics also have many talents and are an extremely heterogeneous group, with many inconsistencies within and among individuals.

Sometimes the talents are as much a component of dyslexia as the struggles. Behavioral Neurologist Norman Geschwind, M.D., refers to what he calls the "special ability hypothesis" in discussing the neurological organization of dyslexia and how it only became a problem in our literate society. He refers to the brain's two hemispheres:

- the left side, which generally controls language and literary functions
- the right side, which generally directs spatial, visual, and creative functions

"If certain changes on the left side of the brain lead to superiority of other regions, particularly on the right side of the brain, then there would be little disadvantage to the carrier of such changes in an illiterate society; their talents would make them highly successful citizens. It isn't surprising then, that this type of brain organization should occur with such high frequency. Only when literacy becomes an important goal is it discovered that a significant fraction of these highly talented individuals suffer from some disadvantage. We are thus brought to the apparently paradoxical notion that the very same anomalies on the left side of the brain that have led to the disability of dyslexia in certain literate societies also determine superiority in some brains. For these reasons, we can speak of a *pathology of superiority* without fear of being contradictory!" (Geschwind 1982, 13-30)

In our literate society, our school system focuses on processing skills typically controlled by the left side of the brain, exacerbating many of the difficulties experienced by dyslexic students. The goal of education should be to help students cope with these issues without losing any of their areas of superiority or decreasing their feelings of self-worth. The following 16 myths about dyslexia seem common among educators and parents. (Note: a complete list of all 16 myths is included on page 29.)

Myth 1	**Fact 1**
Dyslexia only affects reading.	Dyslexia primarily affects reading and spelling. However, the basis of dyslexia is a processing difference. These processing characteristics can affect all aspects of language, resulting in difficulty with listening, speaking, reading comprehension, writing, and some aspects of arithmetic or math. Related processing areas include memory, rapid retrieval, sequencing, spatial awareness, kinesthetic awareness, and figure/ground discrimination.

Myth 2	**Fact 2**
If a person is able to read, he cannot possibly be dyslexic.	Dyslexia is a processing difference resulting from how the brain is organized. Therefore, a dyslexic person remains dyslexic. Many who receive appropriate remediation geared to their processing styles do learn to read, but they remain dyslexic. Even when they learn to read well, their processing differences affect automaticity and efficiency in the higher levels of comprehension or writing. "This deficit . . . is characterized by distinct neurophysiological signature in the left posterior regions of the brain . . ." (Lyon 1995a)

Myth 3	**Fact 3**
Dyslexics can learn to read just like anybody else; they just progress at a slower rate. Therefore, the appropriate remediation is to repeat the same instruction but at a much slower speed.	Dyslexia is a processing difference; dyslexics need to learn to read differently using specific techniques and strategies. Slowly repeating the same material that has not worked will not help a dyslexic develop the appropriate and necessary strategies and skills. That approach merely generates frustration and decreases self-esteem. This reading disability is not a developmental lag; rather, it reflects a persistent deficit (Lyon 1996, 33), indicating that more time or a slower approach will not remediate the problem.

Myth 4	Fact 4
Dyslexics will never learn to read.	Dyslexics can learn to read. A great deal of research, beginning with the pioneering work of Samuel T. Orton in the early part of the 1900s, indicates that dyslexics can and will learn to read if the instructional strategies match their processing needs. Development of phonological awareness is required, along with a multisensory systematic structured language approach, including sound/symbol association, syllable instruction, morphology (base words, roots, affixes), syntax (grammar and language mechanics), and semantics (meaning). Highly replicable research on early reading instruction has demonstrated the mastery in decoding "occurs only when a code-based approach is used to teach that alphabet letters consistently and predictably represent English speech sounds." (Lyon 1996)

Myth 5	Fact 5
Dyslexics struggle with phonics; therefore, phonics should be avoided with these students.	Belief in this myth has probably done more damage to more dyslexics than any other myth! It is true that dyslexic students may have great difficulty with phonics development, particularly traditional phonics. Often, this is due to poor development of the necessary foundation skills in phonological awareness. Research supports and substantiates the need for multisensory phonics in this population of learners, along with a need for development and/or remediation of the phonological processing gaps. "The etiological basis for the deficit word recognition and decoding skills . . . appears to be a specific deficit in phonological processing. Intervention programs that capitalize on code emphasis methodologies are superior to meaning-based language approaches." (Lyon 1995a, 121)

Myth 6

Dyslexia can be diagnosed in a preschool child.

Fact 6

A firm diagnosis of dyslexia is dependent on failure to learn to read. However, risk signs evident in the preschool years may be significant. These include problems in phonological awareness (ability to understand and manipulate sounds), rhyming, word retrieval (dysnomia), sound sequencing, and word sequencing. Articulation may sometimes be a risk sign, especially when combined with other characteristics. However, many young students with poor articulation are not dyslexic.

Myth 7

All dyslexics use mirror writing. Therefore, if a student does not write backwards, he is not dyslexic.

Fact 7

Reversals are developmentally normal through second grade and common within many learning disabilities. Mirror writing, often called the Leonardo Syndrome, after da Vinci, is an extension of reversals and is only one of many visual-spatial characteristics that may be exhibited by some dyslexics. A diagnosis of dyslexia cannot be made based on any single characteristic.

Mirror writing remains relatively rare, and when it exists frequently in a child's work, it may be significant no matter what the age. Delos R. Smith, a dyslexic, states, "I never reversed my letters, but wrote in a perfectly mirrored way." (Rawson 171) Delos, despite intensive remediation by June Orton (wife of Samuel Orton), never overcame his basic natural mirror tendencies. Rather, he made an adjustment to the world around him. (See the anecdote on the left.)

Mirror Music

Delos Smith describes a situation where his tendency for mirror reading/writing became an advantage for him. In music he perceived ascending scales to be descending scales and vice versa. He was quite frustrated with music for seven years until one night when he was tired. He said, "A major change occurred when I tried playing music backwards. I played song after song—Bach, Mozart, anything. I felt no fatigue. I was on an adrenaline high. Euphoria had a new meaning. I was really playing music!" (Pollack 1982, 282)

Myth 8	Fact 8
All dyslexics have very poor writing skills.	There is a wide variety of writing competencies exhibited among dyslexic learners. Some dyslexics are good in both the content and mechanics of writing, with the exception of spelling. Some have extremely good written expression skills but very poor mechanics, or vice versa. Others have difficulties with both aspects of writing. The struggles are due to the organizational aspects of written language and its demands for multi-tasking. A student's struggles are significantly compounded if he experiences the concurrent problem of dysgraphia.

Myth 9	Fact 9
All dyslexics are clumsy, or the converse, all dyslexics are well coordinated.	Coordination is one of the many characteristics which can exist anywhere along a continuum from unskilled to extremely skilled. Many dyslexics may be coordinated in some tasks, but very uncoordinated in others. For example, some students with sloppy, poorly formed letters may be very skilled at constructing puzzles, building with Legos®, and performing other visual-spatial fine motor tasks. Some dyslexics may be clumsy and seem to trip over their own feet. Other dyslexics, such as Bruce Jenner (1976 Olympic Decathlon winner), are very skilled and highly regarded for their athletic abilities.

Myth 10	Fact 10
All dyslexics have a poor sense of direction, or conversely, all dyslexics have a superior directional sense.	This characteristic is another that exists along a continuum from great difficulty to extreme skill. There are some dyslexics who get lost very frequently, even in familiar surroundings. One dyslexic speaker at a Southern California Conference of the Orton Dyslexia Society (now called The International Dyslexia Association) stated, "Even though I have my Ph.D., I still get confused when I park in the parking lot of my own office and will often turn in the wrong direction. This creates much merriment for my colleagues who may be looking out the window." (Thomasson 1993) On the other hand, some dyslexics have a superior sense of direction

Myth 10	**Fact 10,** *continued*
	and only need to be in a location once to develop a strong visual-spatial cognitive map of the location. These individuals often report having an internal sense that it "feels right" to turn in a certain direction when going to a location.

Myth 11	**Fact 11**
All dyslexics have a poor memory, or conversely, all dyslexics have a superior memory.	There are many different aspects of memory, and these typically vary for any individual. Dyslexics can range along a full continuum on any or all of the aspects of memory. In attempting to analyze whether a particular person has a good or poor memory, it is necessary to first define the situation and type of memory being analyzed. Rote sequential memory is typically most difficult for dyslexics, i.e., months of the year, math facts, and spelling. Contextual, experiential, and/or spatial memory may be quite strong.

Myth 12	**Fact 12**
All dyslexics are left-handed.	While many more dyslexics are left-handed, there are also a large number who are right-handed. Research indicates learning disabilities to be 12 times more frequent in left-handers than in right-handed individuals. (Behan and Geschwind 1985)

Myth 13	**Fact 13**
More dyslexics are boys.	The gender ratio in individuals with reading disabilities is no different from the gender ratio in the population as a whole. (Lyon 1996, 33)

Myth 14

Since dyslexia is genetic, if a parent is able to read, the student cannot be dyslexic.

Fact 14

It is true that dyslexia has a genetic base but this myth is false for two reasons: 1) many dyslexics can read and 2) the parent being considered may not represent the genetic link. Some parents may have a dyslexic child due to a genetic link from another relative (aunt, uncle, grandparent), or the parent may be undiagnosed. Studies of monozygotic twins indicate 75-100% concordance of dyslexia, and the frequency of at least one affected first degree relative of identified dyslexic individuals is from 40-70%. (Pennington 1991)

Myth 15

Dyslexics cannot go to college.

Fact 15

Dyslexics can and do succeed in college. Dyslexics are often quite bright and possess many cognitive strengths. Many learn basic skills through a strategies approach focusing on their many intellectual strengths. There is also substantial assistance for students diagnosed as learning disabled, such as extra test time or having a note taker. Because dyslexics process information differently, they perceive the world differently, often leading to great depth of problem solving and creativity.

Myth 16

Dyslexia can be cured.

Fact 16

This is quite false. Dyslexia is a lifelong issue, and although strategies and skills can be taught, the processing components that define dyslexia itself cannot be cured. Many, like Thomas G. West, would not want dyslexia to be cured even if it could be. He discusses the dilemma based on remarks by Geschwind:

> "Not only do many dyslexics carry remarkable talents that benefit their society enormously, but the same talents exist in unusually high frequency among their unaffected relatives. If we could somehow prevent these brain changes, and thus prevent the appearance of dyslexia, might we not find that we have deprived the society of an important and irreplaceable group of individuals endowed with remarkable talents?" (West 1997, 23)

Definition of Dyslexia

A layperson's definition of dyslexia involves letter reversals, such as confusion between *b* and *d*. However, as stated by Sylvia O. Richardson, M.D., past President of IDA, reversal patterns do not diagnose dyslexia. (Richardson 1994) Five- and six-year-old dyslexics may reverse letters or numbers, but this is also true of non-dyslexic children. The difference is that non-dyslexic children begin to correct their errors by age seven or eight, while the dyslexics are delayed in establishing directionality. However, reversals are not the major criteria in identification of dyslexia. The major defining characteristic of dyslexia is specific deficit in the processing of phonological information. In other words, the dyslexic finds it difficult to break the symbol-sound code of the language and to understand the alphabetic principle.

In the mid-1990s, the academic definition of dyslexia and reading disabilities was commonly based on exclusionary language, i.e., what it is not. This provided reliability of basic findings across research programs (Lyon 1995a and 1995b) but it was difficult to operationalize. In 1994, the Orton Dyslexia Society (now IDA) Research Committee constructed a new definition of dyslexia that reduced the exclusionary language and used inclusionary statements, defining dyslexia using current and valid research findings. This definition has been adopted by the National Institute of Child Health and Development (NICHD) for its research programs in dyslexia and learning disabilities.

> Dyslexia is one of several distinct learning disabilities. It is a specific language-based disorder of constitutional origin, characterized by difficulties in single-word decoding, usually reflecting insufficient phonological processing abilities. These difficulties in single-word decoding are often unexpected in relation to age and other cognitive and academic abilities; they are not the result of generalized developmental disability or sensory impairment. Dyslexia is manifested by variable difficulty with different forms of language, often including, in addition to reading problems, a conspicuous problem with acquiring proficiency in writing and spelling. (Lyon 1996, 34)

The more traditional IDA definition is broader than the one above.

> Dyslexia is a neurologically-based, often familial, disorder which interferes with the acquisition and processing of language. Varying in degrees of severity, it is manifested by difficulties in receptive and expressive language—including phonological processing, reading, writing, spelling,

handwriting and sometimes in arithmetic. Dyslexia is not a result of lack of motivation, sensory impairment, inadequate instructional or environmental opportunities, or other limiting conditions, but may occur together with these conditions. Although dyslexia is lifelong, individuals with dyslexia frequently respond successfully to timely and appropriate intervention. (IDA 1998)

Phonological skills play a substantial role related to most prerequisites critical to the development of reading. In speaking (and reading), sounds can be incorrectly added, omitted, substituted, shifted, or repeated. Phonological difficulties provide a significant diagnostic indicator, even in the early preschool years, since the same neurological and genetic factors form the etiological base for both phonological disorders (including articulation) and reading deficiencies.

Phonology refers to the linguistic rules system containing the inventory of speech sounds that occur in language and the rules for combining the sounds into meaningful units. Phonological processing involves the use of phonological information to help the child process first oral, and later written, information. The child's primary task in the early development of reading and spelling is to become aware that speech can be segmented into phonemes (sounds) and that these phonemes represent printed forms. (Liberman 1991, 71) However, many children struggle and do not easily develop the awareness that sounds can be divided into small, discernable segments. This difficulty arises because speech, unlike writing, does not consist of separate phonemes produced one after another in a row over time. Instead, the sounds are co-articulated (overlapped with one another) to permit rapid communication of speech rather than sound by sound production. This property of co-articulation is critical for speech but can be difficult for the beginning reader and speller.

> The advantageous result of co-articulation of speech sounds is that speech can proceed at a satisfactory pace, at a pace, indeed, at which it can be understood. Can you imagine trying to understand speech if it were spelled out to you letter by painful letter? So, co-articulation is certainly advantageous for the perception of speech. But a further result of co-articulation, and a much less advantageous one for the would-be reader, is that there is, inevitably, no neat correspondence between the underlying phonological structure and the sound that comes to the ears. Thus, though the word *bag*, for example, has three phonological units and correspondingly three letters in print, it has only one pulse of sound: the three elements of the underlying phonological

structure—the three phonemes (/b/ /a/ /g/)—have been thoroughly overlapped (co-articulated) into one beginning sound, "bag."

Beginning readers can understand and properly take advantage of the fact that the printed word *bag* has three letters only if they are aware that the spoken word *bag*, with which they are already quite familiar, is divisible into three segments. They will probably not know that spontaneously, because as we have said, there is only one segment of sound, not three, and because the processes of speech perception that recover the phonological structure are automatic and quite unconscious. (Liberman 1991, 5-6)

In addition to serving as a prerequisite for basic reading skills, phonological processing also appears highly related to expressive language development. Similar phonological deficits in both oral and written language are found and children with expressive language disorders (difficulty expressing ideas through language) generally manifest more severe phonological processing difficulties. Children who as preschoolers automatically and naturally play with sounds through rhyming, sound games, and playing with words are demonstrating that they have intuitively learned to process and analyze the phonological system of our language. Children who avoid such games do not develop important and critical prerequisite skills.

Here are some commonly held myths about dyslexia:

1   Dyslexia only affects reading.

2   If a person is able to read, he cannot possibly be dyslexic.

3   Dyslexics can learn to read just like anybody else; they just progress at a slower rate. Therefore, the appropriate remediation is to repeat the same instruction but at a much slower speed.

4   Dyslexics will never learn to read.

5   Dyslexics struggle with phonics; therefore, phonics should be avoided with these students.

6   Dyslexia can be diagnosed in a preschool child.

7   All dyslexics use mirror writing. Therefore, if a student does not write backwards, he is not dyslexic.

8   All dyslexics have very poor writing skills.

9   All dyslexics are clumsy, or the converse, all dyslexics are well coordinated.

10   All dyslexics have a poor sense of direction, or conversely, all dyslexics have a superior directional sense.

11   All dyslexics have a poor memory, or conversely, all dyslexics have a superior memory.

12   All dyslexics are left-handed.

13   More dyslexics are boys.

14   Since dyslexia is genetic, if a parent is able to read, the student cannot be dyslexic.

15   Dyslexics cannot go to college.

16   Dyslexia can be cured.

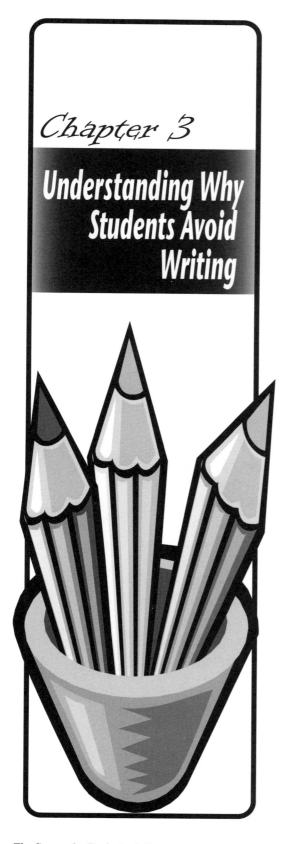

Chapter 3

Understanding Why Students Avoid Writing

Many students today dislike the writing process or avoid it altogether. For some, writing is a very laborious task because there are so many subcomponents that need to be pulled together. For others, the reason lies in some processing difficulties, such as dyslexia or dysgraphia. And some students simply feel writing takes too long. Some educators wonder if students no longer enjoy the slower, more refined process of written communication because they spend so much time watching the faster-paced visual modality of television.

Students with learning problems, even those who read well, frequently submit written work that is brief and/or difficult to read. Such students can be victims of misunderstandings, a problem that becomes much more pronounced at the secondary level. "Accusations of laziness, poor motivation, and a reprehensible attitude are often directed toward deficit writers. The results can be a serious loss of incentive—a generalized academic disenchantment and demoralization." (Levine 1998, 363)

Here are some reasons students might avoid writing:

- They have a hard time getting started and feel overwhelmed by the task.
- Forming letters isn't an automatic process; they have to concentrate.
- They struggle to organize and use mechanics of writing.
- They are slow and inefficient in retrieving the right word(s) to express an idea.
- They struggle to develop their ideas fluently.
- They struggle to keep track of their thoughts while also getting them down on paper.
- They feel that the process of writing on paper is slow and tedious.

- They feel that their papers never turn out the way they want.

- They realize that their papers are still sloppy even though they spent substantial time and effort on their attempts.

- They are dysgraphic, which causes multiple struggles at the basic processing levels.

- They are dyslexic, which causes very poor spelling and interferes with automatic use of writing mechanics.

As parents and teachers, we can help students deal with their lack of enjoyment of the writing process. We can also assist with their poor skill development. The techniques are twofold. Students need to:

- develop a greater understanding of and appreciation for the purpose of writing

- develop more efficient skills

When students have a combination of this understanding and the skills they need, they can then apply techniques and abilities in a wide range of situations. This is especially true and necessary for dyslexic and/or dysgraphic students who are compensating for many processing inefficiencies in the language domain.

Understanding the Purpose of Writing

It is important for a five- to seven-year-old child to understand that writing is speech written down. However, the student needs to progress past that level to recognize the differences between spoken and written language. In today's society, spoken language often contains multiple, incomplete sentences and slang expressions. These changes are frequently and easily accepted; however, such usage should stay within the spoken domain. Slang and many common oral expressions do not belong in technical written language. There are many ways to clarify the spoken word (expression, vocal inflections, body language, visual stimuli) that are not available when dealing with the written word. The written word depends on structure, clarity of expression, and awareness of the reader's needs. When these elements are missing, writing deteriorates and the message becomes unclear.

Students learn to speak by listening to and practicing language. They learn to write by reading and practicing writing. This process is facilitated when they have confidence in and are excited by the writing process. Strategies generated by using a variety of modalities enhance the prewriting stages and help students focus on writing to achieve a purpose. Multiple strategies are useful to make writing seem less like drudgery and more like a fun, engrossing activity. As writing becomes more relevant and more exciting, students will use it more, increasing their experience and practice.

Throughout their school careers, students need a multiplicity of guided writing experiences. Many students, whether or not they have a learning difficulty, do not know how to proceed step-by-step through their written material and often consider their first drafts to be close to or the same as their final drafts. Their writing experiences should start simply, but build to more complex activities. Incorporating fun within the activities will help the students develop skills while simultaneously building confidence.

Skill Development

A strong foundation is necessary for the development of writing efficiency. This base is provided by underlying processing skills, and the stronger the base, the more solid and automatic the child's development will be. Difficulties in processing at this level suggest a dysgraphic pattern. The mechanical and content skills which follow are dependent upon a strong foundation in basic processing. These skills need to be in place so the student can then advance to the level of writing efficiency. Figure 3.1 illustrates the relationship between mechanical and content skills as they relate to writing efficiency.

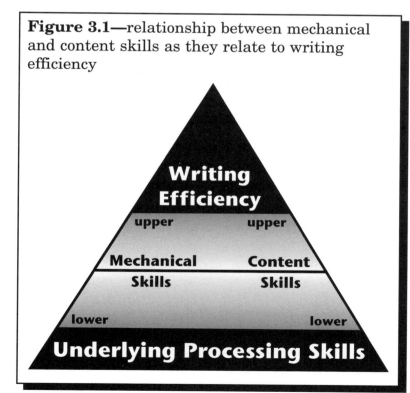

Figure 3.1—relationship between mechanical and content skills as they relate to writing efficiency

These levels are important because each provides a stepping stone upon which future levels are built. If the foundation or any level is inconsistent and metaphorically made of sand, the top level will sag and frequently collapse. Students who have difficulty with writing need remediation and/or support consisting of bypass strategies and compensations.

The process of writing consists of many subskills. As these are acquired and become more automatic, each level then becomes more solid. Automaticity at each level is essential because it allows the student to attempt more cognitively difficult skills or techniques at each stage. When a student becomes overloaded at any level, automaticity is decreased. Automaticity does not mean that a student must have perfect skills, such as grammar, spelling, or punctuation, and it is not the same as mastery of a given skill. Automaticity indicates that a student is able to perform automatically, demonstrating a level of proficiency and ease of performance which will allow him to integrate skills and progress in writing development.

Underlying Processing Skills

The box on the right contains a list of underlying processing skills essential to writing. Problems in any of these skills will cause a student to struggle with writing, whether or not he is technically dysgraphic. All dysgraphic students struggle with at least some of these areas, but as with all areas of struggle, no student has all the difficulties listed. The following discussion identifies the range of possibilities as well as how each component interrelates with others.

✔ physical components of writing

✔ speed of motor performance

✔ efficient motor patterns

✔ automatic motor memory

✔ automaticity of performances

✔ active working memory

✔ language formulation and ideation

✔ awareness of metacognitive strategies.

Physical components of writing

Students must first master the physical, or motor, components of writing in order to eventually retrieve the motor patterns required for writing letters quickly and efficiently. This process begins with recognizing and producing a specific shape, which is a complex task of sequencing involving a series of steps. To master the physical components of writing, the student must develop these skills:

- ability to use a tool (pencil or crayon) to exert appropriate force and movement within specific spatial limitations
- ability to plan and control movement with acceptable speed and fluency
- ability to perform fine motor movements reciprocally and make directional changes fluently, easily, and automatically, including the ability to stop at a given point on command

These steps represent important prerequisites for all of the other underlying processing skills.

Speed of motor performance

Motor movements need to be made smoothly and with good speed. Some students may be very slow in making letter forms due to reduced speed of their motor performances; they are slow in forming each of the lines necessary to create a form or a letter. This could be related to a processing difficulty such as dysgraphia, poor pencil control, or the manner in which the letter form was taught to the child. Some children who are self-taught regarding letter form never develop the skills to consistently and automatically make each letter in the most efficient manner. Some children do not form a good mental image of what they are trying to write. They may have a blueprint for the action but experience difficulty implementing it motorically. (Levine 1998, 209) Consequently, their writing is slow and awkward, and they have serious difficulty with performance. Such children may write with as much space between letters as there is between words.

Efficient motor patterns

When first learning a new motor skill, we watch our movements carefully and make many readjustments as our movements begin to match our idea of the desired movement. This idea of the desired movement is often in the form of a visualized image, sometimes visual, sometimes kinesthetic, and often a combination. When we repeat the sequence of movements many times, it begins to feel familiar and builds a pattern. As our memory establishes this pattern firmly, it then becomes automatic. We perform automatic skills easily, with little or no conscious attention to the component parts, and with little or no effort required to retrieve the kinesthetic image.

A common example of developing such a motor pattern is when a 16-year-old first learns to drive a car. Initially, she pays attention and makes conscious choices to direct every movement. She might say, "The key goes in here, gas pedal is there," etc. As the skills become more automatic, the student's mind is free to focus on other activities rather than only the primary motor activity involved. As automaticity develops, the young driver can play the radio or carry on a conversation while driving. These activities generally can't be performed until driving becomes automatic. Similarly, an adult driving a carload of noisy children may not be bothered by the noise until a problem appears in the road ahead. At that point, the adult may need quiet and may demand silence to enhance his concentration.

As is common when learning any complex motor movement, students rely heavily on visual information and conscious decisions as they learn to write letters and numbers. They correct letters or parts of letters that do not look right and their performance is slow, deliberate, and hesitant. When letter formation is stuck at this level, the student is unable to develop efficient motor patterns.

Automatic motor memory

Memory is a critical component for learning and performing complex motor skills. To perform automatic movements, we need internal information from joints and muscles, an awareness that develops with age and experience. Although students begin with substantial conscious decisions about letter form, by the end of first grade or the beginning of second grade, most rely more on internal feedback related to their images of the form. At this point, their writing speed accelerates and copying becomes easier. When kinesthetic imagery is used for guidance, the child can use smooth letter formation even when her eyes shift to the material being copied. The child knows how the movements feel when making a letter and can repeat the sequence using mostly internal cues, making continual matches with the internal image of the form. Each part of the sequence is cued by the previous movement, and the process proceeds automatically. Vision is used for fine-tuning corrections and spatial placement. From fourth through seventh grade, motor patterns for letter and number formations become firmly established as writing becomes more fluent and automatic. In the classroom, as the amount of written work increases, the demand grows for quick retrieval of automatic movement patterns for writing.

A child with weak motor memory does not consistently recall the correct sequence of movements needed to form letters. Consistency is a key factor because her memory fluctuates; sometimes a letter is easily recalled and other times it is not. Copying is an extremely laborious task because she needs to attend to the form while making the letter rather than just the visual information she is copying.

Automaticity of performances

Many aspects might interfere with the development of automatic performances. An overload of either cognitive or attentional factors contributes to a variety of writing difficulties for children who attempt writing at levels that are higher than their cognitive and linguistic abilities are able to support. When students are in overload, their writing seems to greatly decrease in maturity; they do not use, or incorrectly use, skills which appeared to have been learned. For example, a student may be able to correctly punctuate sentences in a list but does not use periods when writing a paragraph. Students with dyslexia or dysgraphia are in a predicament because they lack automaticity with lower level skills, such as letter formation, directionality, sound/symbol relationships, and early spelling patterns. This lack of automaticity almost ensures cognitive and attentional overload within the writing process. Such students are frequently able to verbally tell a story at a much higher level than they can write a similar story. While many students may demonstrate such a difference, the difference is much more discrepant for these students because of the influence of their learning problems on grammatical structure, automaticity, formulation, spelling, and mechanics.

Active working memory

Active working memory is the ability to hold information in mind while manipulating or working on that information. It permits the process which occurs between input of the pattern and the output, or response. It is similar to multitasking on a computer; the computer needs sufficient memory to be able to hang onto all the parts and switch back and forth easily and efficiently. Reduced active working memory can be observed in the student who struggles to organize a task but then loses pieces of the task while involved in its completion.

The writing process is a very complex activity wherein the student needs to simultaneously focus on many different aspects of writing mechanics and content. Effective active working memory is essential when writing; the student must remember what he is writing, find the right vocabulary, connect his ideas, and simultaneously use correct mechanics. The weaker the student's active working memory, the greater his chances of experiencing overload during the writing process.

There are many factors that can help increase active working memory for a student. One component is to increase efficiency and automaticity of each subskill. Then the student can employ specific strategies to hang onto the components. Each student needs to be helped to find his own particular combination of strategies to increase active working memory within the writing activity. You can use the writing strategies in Part Two of this book to help a student increase his active working memory.

Language formulation and ideation

Formulation is the ability to put words together to express a desired idea while maintaining acceptable grammar, word order, a logical flow of ideas, and pronunciation (in speech) or spelling (in writing). Ideation involves the ability to convert an idea which is more global or general into a form that can be communicated to others. Formulation and ideation can be verbal or written. A student with adequate skills in these areas is usually able to create sentences (and paragraphs) that communicate and explain the intended meaning in a fairly fluent, concise manner.

Many students with difficulties in these processing areas struggle to get started. While they have multiple ideas floating around in their heads, they cannot pull them together, organize them, and decide upon a starting point. Some students have difficulty generating ideas in the first place, even when cues are given. As these students struggle to pull together the ideas related to their topics, their difficulties may become quite pronounced. Such students may create excuses as they are to begin their writing, such as sharpening their pencils three or four times. A student who experiences these problems becomes very frustrated because by the time he begins his first sentence, the rest of the class might be finished with the assignment. This type of experience decreases a student's enthusiasm for participating in writing activities.

Awareness of metacognitive strategies

It is common for students with weak skills in language-based activities, especially writing, to have a weakness in metacognition. Such students have been termed *inactive learners.* (Torgesen 1982, 455) These students struggle to use active strategies, and they lack knowledge about the ways in which they think. Because of this, they have trouble regulating their learning and rarely monitor themselves. They are unable to step back and conceptualize the learning processes needed to meet the demands of the task. This poor metacognitive awareness makes it hard for them to know when they are going astray or when they need to self-correct. (Levine 1998, 232)

Within the writing process, students need to understand how each skill relates to other skills, when to employ various skills, and how the skills need to be integrated to function as a whole. All students, but especially those with learning disabilities, need to become specifically aware of the subskills and strategies needed to write. This awareness is important as well as an ability to employ self-regulation skills such as planning, evaluation, and self-checking. A metacognitive approach to written expression and study strategies is useful to learning content or procedures. For the student with dyslexia or dysgraphia, such an approach is both useful and essential. Metacognitive awareness is often the best connection between learning disability and learning ability.

Mechanical Skills

Mechanical skills that influence writing are divided into lower and upper level skills, as indicated in the box on the right. The lower level mechanical skills involve using a pencil as a tool and being able to develop consistent use of form and space when writing letters, including automatic letter form. When a student uses erratic writing or inconsistent letter form, he does not receive appropriate feedback to reinforce a consistent motor pattern for each letter. Other skills, such as spelling, punctuation, and capitalization are then compromised, primarily because too much cognitive energy is placed on the motor aspects of writing.

As the mechanical components for forming letters become more automatic, the student is able to use the pencil more efficiently as a tool and write letters using consistent form and space, with letter form being automatic. Mel Levine calls this graphomotor facility the combination of factors which include an ease with the mechanical aspects of writing. This is the most conspicuous fine-motor achievement for school-aged children. (Levine 1987, 216)

Before students can easily progress into higher level mechanics, they need to develop skill in other lower-level basic skills, such as punctuation, capitalization, and spelling. Complete

Lower Level Mechanics

✔ Use of pencil as a tool

✔ Consistent use of form and space when writing letters

✔ Automatic letter form

✔ Punctuation

✔ Capitalization

✔ Spelling

Upper Level Mechanics

✔ Automaticity of lower level skills

✔ Integration of lower level skills with content

✔ Grammar

✔ Semantics (clear and appropriate word usage)

✔ Speed of motor performances

✔ Clarity, precision, and confidence evident in the written product

skill development in each of these areas is not required. However, there should be enough automaticity to allow the student to proceed without stopping his flow of ideas in order to figure out how to create a given letter or where to place a period.

Spelling is often the most difficult area. A student needs enough automaticity to write a representation of the word that allows him to recognize it when he returns to proofread his paper. This is a critical aspect for dyslexic students, for whom spelling remains a problem throughout their careers.

Moving into upper level mechanics enables many students to begin to enjoy writing. Once the basic lower level mechanical skills are somewhat automatic, the student can attend more to content, and consequently, grow in skill and efficiency. Upper level mechanics include more sophisticated use of sentence structure, punctuation, and spelling. As these skills develop, the student has greater freedom to attend to content. At this point, the student should have enough fluency and grammatical knowledge to automatically use basic grammatical components without extensive pauses to think about them. Even advanced writers occasionally stop to think about a specific verb form or grammatical consistency; however, the basics of grammar need to be automatic.

Semantics, which involves clear and appropriate word usage, should also be at a fairly automatic and fluent level. The student who writes, "I saw the stuff and put it over by the thing, next to that over there," does not present a clear message. Frequent use of nonspecific referents may be a clue to reduced semantics and/or difficulties with automatic word retrieval. When the student efficiently uses upper level mechanics, he will be able to integrate the lower level functions and skills with content and then write with clarity, precision, confidence, and, ideally, with some enjoyment.

In Eli's writing samples (Figures 1.1 and 1.2 on pages 13-14), you can see he never reached automaticity in the mechanical skills. Consequently, when he attempted to pull in these skills (as required by his teachers), his content decreased, as did his love of story writing. This love was never rekindled and represents an educational disservice to this creative student.

Content Skills

Content skills related to writing involve both lower and upper level skills, as listed in the box. These begin with basic, clear organization and expression of ideas and progress into more mature skills that can be flexibly used with enthusiasm, clarity, and purpose.

Writing efficiency: a developmental process using the content skills

Efficiency in the mechanical aspects leads to development of greater skill in expressing ideas in a written form. It takes years to learn the basics of grammar, spelling, vocabulary, and ideation before being able to write a simple multi-part story or efficiently explain concepts and ideas. Mel Levine views writing as "... the final common pathway, the merger of multiple development functions." (Levine 1987, 308) He believes it to be the most critical academic output skill for children in the middle and upper elementary grades. The chart on page 45 presents the first four of Levine's seven stages of writing. (Levine 1987, 310) These initial stages are related to typical educational expectations and perceptual-motor development through the elementary and middle school years.

Writing is a process of integrating developmental functions. What we see on the paper (the cursive or manuscript print) is the end product of this process. In the primary grades, good writing is synonymous with neat and organized work. By fourth grade, the emphasis shifts to the structure and content of the writing, i.e., vocabulary, syntax, and grammar. In the seventh grade and thereafter, formal writing becomes more linguistically complex than speaking. At that level, students are expected to frequently synthesize and develop ideas using written prose. Following is a summary of various aspects of writing that students acquire through grade levels, as related to Levine's seven stages:

Lower Level Content Skills

✔ Formulating ideas

✔ Organizing ideas

✔ Representing ideas with clarity and in sequence

Upper Level Content Skills

✔ Writing using different writing styles

✔ Being flexible in the writing process

✔ Understanding the viewpoint of the reader

✔ Using writing as a vehicle through which thoughts are discovered and developed

✔ Using writing as a personal search for meaning in a reflective way

✔ Writing with enthusiasm

Imitation: The imitation stage of writing is critical and an important part of development in preschool and kindergarten. At this level, the child mimics writing and is beginning to acquire the ability to form letters and numbers. The mechanical aspect of learning to hold a pencil or crayon correctly is very important at this stage.

Graphic Presentation: In first and second grades, graphic presentation becomes more critical. The student learns more about mechanical skills, such as form, spacing, capitalization, and spelling. It is important at this stage for the student to learn to form letters faster and with a beginning degree of automaticity. Many students become excited as they discover the conventions of spacing, punctuation, and capitalization. Students with dysgraphia often have substantial problems at this stage of development.

Progressive Incorporation: Toward the end of second grade and continuing through fourth grade, students enter the stage of progressive incorporation. At this stage they progressively incorporate more functions and skills within their writing. They begin to use upper level mechanics and lower level content skills. Students become aware of writing as a process of communicating, but generally their written language is much less sophisticated than their spoken language. There is very little pre-planning to writing at this stage.

Automization: Generally, beginning in fourth grade and continuing through seventh grade, students' skills reach more automization, especially of the mechanical aspects regarding written form, space, grammar, spelling, capitalization, and punctuation. It is essential for students to have good motor memory and automatic letter form so that they can write with less conscious effort, placing more emphasis on planning and communication of ideas.

Elaboration: During the middle school years, students enter the stage of elaboration, where they begin to use writing to establish and express a viewpoint. At this point in development, their written language should exceed the complexity of their everyday speech. Therefore, students at this level tend to develop greater sophistication in language through their experiences with both reading and writing. It is important for students to learn to summarize through writing and to be able to integrate information from multiple sources. They begin appropriately using connective words other than *and* and words and phrases such as *therefore, finally,* and *for example* to establish transition between their ideas. Students with difficulties in reading miss out on a valuable source of language learning, unless they are frequently read to using age-appropriate materials.

Personalization Diversification: Beginning in the high school years, students should be developing more independent, sophisticated writing. Levine calls this stage *personalization diversification*. Students need to become aware that there are different styles of writing and that different styles are used for different purposes. Good writers understand that writing is never quite finished. Further discussion and editing can always strengthen or clarify a piece. Good writers know that good writing does not happen in one draft, and that they must be patient to produce their best work.

Epistemic Writing: The highest level of writing occurs when writing integrates reflective thought. Writing can then be used for a personal search for meaning. It is no longer merely a means of conveying thoughts, but rather a vehicle through which thoughts are discovered and developed. This process, called *epistemic writing*, remains out of reach for many students. In today's society, many do not reach this level of writing until after several years of college experience, if then. Although occasionally students reach this level while in high school or beginning college years, this level of achievement is becoming more rare.

The different stages of writing development are based on the cognitive processes and the writing skills of each previous level. As a student progresses through the continuum, his writing skill and sophistication increases. By understanding the basic mechanical and content components of writing within the framework of normal development, a teacher is better able to identify what is appropriate and inappropriate for students at a particular grade level. It is difficult, if not impossible, to identify what is not appropriate unless one knows the related developmental hierarchy. With that knowledge, it is possible to identify where a student needs additional help. Through use of multisensory strategies, it is often easier to encourage the needed extra practice that students may not readily accept using other methodologies.

Overall Guidelines

There are many reasons students may avoid writing, but most relate to the concept that writing is not fun or enjoyable. When writing is not meaningful, it is difficult to pull together the variety of skills needed to develop enthusiasm about writing. Students learn to write by writing, which then gives them the confidence to continue to write and continue to develop their skills. Using a variety of modalities can help create the enthusiasm for writing and help students view writing as a more meaningful activity.

It is also important to analyze the lower level skills to ensure that students have appropriately developed automaticity in these skills. When students are frustrated with individual components related to the task of writing and/or when they struggle to get started or to keep track of their thoughts, then the writing process is not fun and their lack of enthusiasm becomes evident. Writing remains at the level of drudgery no matter how exciting the topics, and students may feel threatened by the process of writing.

The goal for these students is to reduce the frustration, struggles, and threatening feelings. Increasing automaticity of skills is required to increase overall writing automaticity for a student. When automaticity, as developed by metacognitive awareness of the writing process and use of specific strategies, is combined with skill development and bypass strategies, the student should be able to deal with the vast majority of written expression tasks. The next step is to integrate purpose and meaning to generate fun and lead to enthusiasm for writing.

Levine's First 4 Stages of Writing

Stage/Grade	Typical Educational Expectations	Perceptual-Motor Development	Characteristics
Imitation (Preschool-Kindergarten)	• Coloring, tracing, and copying leads to mastery of most forms and some manuscript letters	• Hand preference develops • Stability in arm and wrist lays foundation for fine-motor skill • Brief attention needed • Reversals and associated mouth movements common	• Excited with pre-writing • Attempts to mimic true writing • Acquires letter and number forms • Begins to appreciate spelling • Uses invented spellings
Graphic Presentation (Grade 1-Beginning 2)	• Mastery of upper- and lowercase manuscript • Understands spacing and capitalization • Learns to spell and use one- to two-syllable words • Emphasis on mechanics and expressing ideas	• Hand dominance and pencil grip established • Begins to rely on internal feedback to form letters faster • Mouth movements still common • Reversals lessen	• Concerned with visual appearances • Uses spacing and capitalization • Fine motor control increases • Spelling ability increases • Language use unsophisticated
Progressive Incorporation (End Grade 2-Grade 4)	• Content simple and spontaneous • Emphasis on capitalization, syntax, and punctuation • Introduction of cursive	• Reversals and mouth movements uncommon • Recognizes mistakes through increased visual discrimination	• Is aware of writing as a process • Integrates mechanics (punctuation, capitalization) with language (morphology, syntax, narrative, organization) • Written language is less sophisticated than speech • Little emphasis on pre-planning • Begins to rewrite
Automization (Grades 4-7)	• Volume of writing increases with attention to spelling, vocabulary, and grammar • Emphasis on development of ideas	• Motor memory essential for automatic letter production • Active working memory is needed for processing simultaneous sensory input, motor output, and language	• Writes with less conscious effort • Capacity to write and think increases • Attains cursive writing fluency • Is able to produce larger volumes of writing • Written language begins to approximate verbal levels of maturity • Places greater emphasis on planning and draft writing

Chapter 4

Symptoms of Dyslexia

Learning disabilities refer to a heterogeneous group of difficulties in acquiring and using skills for listening, speaking, reading, writing, reasoning, or math. Dyslexia refers to the cluster of language-based skills related to reading, spelling, and writing. Because of its base in language, it may also affect listening and speaking in varying degrees, from hardly at all to severely.

The difficulties experienced by a dyslexic involve a processing difference which is intrinsic and occurs across the life span. The resultant reading difficulties reflect a persistent deficit and are not a developmental lag. This means that these children do not tend to catch up if given more time or presented with material repeated in a slower manner. These children need a different type of learning so they can compensate for their processing difficulties.

Researchers have conducted longitudinal studies wherein they follow children for many years to determine what aspects predict reading disabilities at high-school age. Such longitudinal studies indicate that of children with reading disabilities in the third grade, 74% will still have disabilities in ninth grade. (Fletcher et al 1993; Francis et al 1994; Shaywitz et al 1992) These figures are outstanding as well as frightening. As more parents, teachers, and other professionals increase their understanding of these processing patterns, we can hope that these figures will change.

Individuals with reading difficulties differ from one another and from typical readers along an entire continuum rather than being organized into one or two clearly defined groupings. Consequently, early attempts at subtyping have not proven fruitful. Dyslexia is a lifelong disability representing a difference in brain organization. Research is beginning to suggest that the brains of dyslexics reorganize and learn to compensate for the reading disability by using other parts of the brain. The angular gyrus (Figure 4.1 on page 48) is an area in the back of the brain which sits at the junction of three brain regions that regulate vision, sensory, and emotional information (the occipital, temporal, and parietal lobes). The angular gyrus is an important pathway in processing the sight and sound information that enables people to understand what is being read. Normally, there is a complex two-way communication between the left angular gyrus and the other areas which are utilized to process visual and auditory information related to reading. A study by Barry Horwitz and Judith Rumsey (National Institute of Mental Health) indicated that dyslexic men, even though they learn to read, did not make any of the functional connections in the left angular gyrus that normal readers make. "They are not using the same networks; they have found other ways to compensate." (reported by Jamie Talan, *Newsday* July 29, 1998, A24) This study provides substantial prognostic optimism (a term first used by Samuel T. Orton): dyslexics can learn to read beyond pure compensatory techniques, such as books on tape.

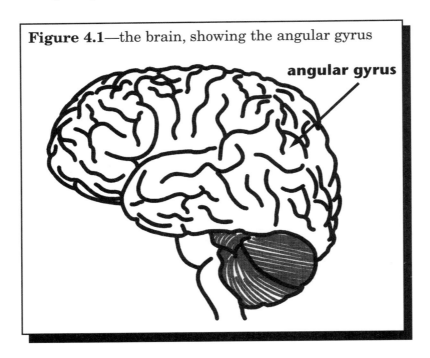

Figure 4.1—the brain, showing the angular gyrus

angular gyrus

Many symptoms accompany dyslexia. It is important to recognize that each dyslexic student is different from every other dyslexic student. A single dyslexic individual will not demonstrate all of the symptoms, nor does any one symptom indicate dyslexia. Each symptom represents an aspect of normal development; but in the dyslexic, the symptom often persists past the time when it is normally integrated into the system. Each dyslexic differs from other dyslexics because these characteristics exist in different combinations and varying degrees of impact. The symptoms are listed on the next page by category.

Symptoms related to dyslexia:

Oral Language	Written Language	Other
❏ Delayed spoken language	❏ Difficulty decoding words; identifying words in isolation or in content	❏ Confusion about directions in space or time (*right/left, early/late, months/days, yesterday/tomorrow*)
❏ Poor awareness of sounds in words: sound order, rhymes, or sequence of syllables (may or may not affect articulation)	❏ Omission of word endings or small words when reading	❏ Difficulty with calendar or clock concepts
❏ Inability to produce rhyming words by elementary school age	❏ Difficulty encoding words—spelling	❏ Confusion regarding prepositions (*on/off, up/down, under/over*)
❏ Imprecise or incomplete interpretation of language that is heard	❏ Reversals and inversions of letters and numbers, e.g., *b/d, p/q, n/u,* 2/5, 6/9	❏ Difficulty with rote automatic recall (such as math facts)
❏ Word retrieval struggles	❏ Poor sequencing of numbers or letters, e.g., *sing/sign, left/felt, soiled/solid,* 12/21	❏ Difficulty in math—often related to sequencing of steps, directionality, or to the language of mathematics
❏ Difficulty fluently expressing thoughts orally, especially when language is requested on demand	❏ Persistent difficulty with oral reading	❏ Excessive daydreaming or especially active imagination
	❏ Problems with reading comprehension, especially at higher levels	❏ Confusion about right- or left-handedness
	❏ Difficulty with handwriting	❏ Unusual difficulty learning a foreign language
	❏ Difficulty expressing thoughts in written form	❏ Similar problems among relatives

It is important to remember that no single symptom characterizes dyslexia. A given individual will exhibit a cluster of symptoms, with each person's cluster differing from every other person's cluster.

Processing Strengths and Weaknesses

Within many areas, dyslexics can have both processing strengths and difficulties. They may struggle to process written language regarding the mechanics of handwriting, syntax, or spelling, but they may also have an extreme strength in their ability to be creative and paint a picture with words. Each dyslexic is different, and because of this, each individual demonstrates variations within his strengths and/or weaknesses. The following chart identifies some general processing strengths and weaknesses that may be exhibited by people with dyslexia.

Processing Area	Observable Phenomena Indicating Difficulties	Observable Phenomena Indicating Strengths
Phonological processing, specifically phonological awareness	Ability to: ✔ Segment sentences into words ✔ Segment words into syllables ✔ Segment syllables into sounds ✔ Manipulate sounds within syllables and words ✔ Rhyme words ✔ Concentrate with background noise (figure/ground)	Rarely observed
Written language	✔ Handwriting (form) ✔ Spelling ✔ Written syntax ✔ Vocabulary retrieval ✔ Use of discourse in writing ✔ Decreased writing speed	✔ Handwriting (form) ✔ Creativity ✔ Content and ideas ✔ Ability to *paint* a picture with words ✔ Ability to *persuade* with words
Metacognitive processes	Automatic organization skills in: ✔ Planning ✔ Self-monitoring ✔ Self-evaluation ✔ Self-modification ✔ Sequential procedures	Development of strategies in: ✔ Planning ✔ Self-monitoring ✔ Self-evaluation ✔ Self-modification ✔ Sequential procedures

Processing Area	Observable Phenomena Indicating Difficulties	Observable Phenomena Indicating Strengths
Vocabulary	✔ Word retrieval: words get *stuck* (dysnomia) ✔ Tendency to substitute words ✔ Use of non-specific referents (*thing, stuff*)	✔ Vocabulary knowledge ✔ Use of high-level words ✔ Comprehension of complex concepts ✔ Ability to quickly substitute a word when desired word gets *stuck*
Receptive language (interpretation)	✔ Understanding and processing language information, especially as the chunk size and complexity increases ✔ Interpretation of slang in social situations ✔ Understanding abstractions	✔ Nonverbal communication, i.e., nonverbal messages; astute awareness of hidden messages ✔ Efficient and skilled listening ✔ Understanding abstractions and slang
Expressive language	✔ Organizing ideas verbally ✔ Explaining ideas verbally, especially spontaneously ✔ Word and grammar usage ✔ Articulation ✔ Language-based social skills	✔ Speaking skills, especially with prior preparation ✔ Verbal explanations and elaborations ✔ Use of language for comedy, persuasion, or creativity
Math	✔ Some of the same processing problems for reading are at the root of math struggles ✔ Arithmetic: automatic facts, computation procedures ✔ Confusion regarding language terms ✔ Nonverbal problem solving and concept formation	✔ High level understanding of spatial components dealing with numbers ✔ Conceptual understanding related to math and numbers

Processing Area	Observable Phenomena Indicating Difficulties	Observable Phenomena Indicating Strengths
Visual interpretations	✔ Figure ground: finding an object on a crowded background; finding a person in a crowded room ✔ Visual skill inefficiencies involving eye movements and teaming: tracking, saccades, focusing ✔ Quick automatic visual interpretation	✔ Construction and organization of clear charts, graphs, drawings ✔ Constructing puzzles ✔ Small object manipulation (i.e., Legos®) ✔ Excellent awareness and recall of details in environment ✔ Astute awareness of details related to people (See Figure 4.2 on page 53.)
Spatial and bodily kinesthetic areas	✔ Converting sequential visual information into a motor format (letters, direct copying) ✔ Fine motor skills: poor writing ✔ Gross motor skills: klutzy ✔ Getting lost even in a familiar environment	✔ Construction skills and manipulation of small objects ✔ Higher-level construction skills (i.e., 3-D puzzles) ✔ Ability to easily find way around environment ✔ Skilled coordination
Attention	✔ Disorders can coexist with dyslexia ✔ Strong tendency for daydreaming	✔ Intense concentration on a task

Early Indicators of Risk for Dyslexia

Typically, dyslexia is not identified or diagnosed until school age. At that time one can determine whether or not the child actually has difficulty acquiring the code system for English as represented by written language. Many states require a significant discrepancy to exist in identifying a learning disability, and therefore, children may not even be tested until second or third grade. However, there are many high risk signs that can be adequately observed even at the preschool level. It is of great benefit to be on the lookout for such signs, especially in a child who has a family history of dyslexia. If these signs are noted, then intervention can be initiated that will facilitate the child's learning once he gets to school. The label is not important; enhancing the child's developmental efficiency is much more important.

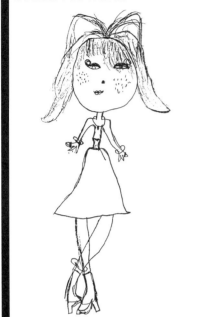

Figure 4.2—drawing by a dyslexic girl who at age 7-2 can't rhyme, use inventive spelling, or sound out words

Early intervention is especially important because the basis for a child's difficulties with word recognition and decoding skills has been shown to be a specific deficit in phonological processing. The importance of preschool language acquisition to later academic achievement is well documented. (Wallach and Butler 1994) This includes strong evidence that a preschooler's ability to follow directions is reflected in facility to develop reading, writing, and spelling skills during the school years. (Butler 1988, 44)

Caution is advised in using the following at-risk symptoms. The list is not meant to identify whether any particular individual will or will not have significant reading and spelling problems intrinsic to dyslexia. Rather, the list should be used to identify clusters of symptoms in children. When a given child demonstrates a cluster, it would be prudent to provide extra assistance as early as possible to help the child fill in missing prerequisite skills. This will provide the individual with the greatest possible start in the reading process whether or not the child is dyslexic. If, however, the child is dyslexic, providing an extra head start will be all the more advantageous. Perhaps in the future, technology will advance to where a low-cost, non-invasive medical test will indicate brain reorganization patterns characteristic of dyslexia. In the meantime, as educators and parents, it is prudent to look at symptoms and deal with them in the most advantageous way without labeling preschoolers and other young children as dyslexic.

Here are some high risk symptoms that may indicate a future problem in development of reading and writing skills:

- ❏ Late development of talking compared to age peers
- ❏ Articulation difficulties: child cannot make sounds expected at his age. For example: inability to use /d/ or /t/ sound by age 4½ or 5; difficulty saying blends, as /sp/ in *spoon* at age five or six; or omission of sounds in familiar words
- ❏ Persistent difficulties with sequencing of sounds within words. Example: "gispetti" for *spaghetti* or "runroader" for *roadrunner*
- ❏ Continuance of what seems to be baby talk, such as "ninimun" for *minimum*, "buff cuttons" for *cuff buttons*
- ❏ Difficulty following directions at a level similar to age peers
- ❏ Irregular language development, e.g., the child's talking does not sound like his peers in terms of word order, grammar, or word usage
- ❏ Great difficulty learning the names of colors

- ❏ Great difficulty learning the names of shapes
- ❏ Great difficulty learning the names of letters
- ❏ A struggle to learn nursery rhymes
- ❏ Extensive slurring of words when memorizing nursery rhymes or singing the alphabet
- ❏ Avoidance or lack of enjoyment of rhyming and/or inability to recognize whether two words rhyme
- ❏ Avoidance of playing with words, i.e., making up their own words or rhyming words, especially in stories
- ❏ Difficulty recognizing sound similarities. For example: onset tasks—when given three words, only two of which start with the same letter, child can identify the word that starts with a different sound (cup, cut, *fun*)
- ❏ Inability to create a story based on picture clues
- ❏ Confusion about simple directional terms such as *up* and *down*

Vignettes: What Do Dyslexic Symptoms Look Like In Real People?

1. *Scott Adams, creator of Dilbert cartoon, on creativity*

Scott demonstrates substantial creativity and feels that some (if not most) of his creativity is due to the difference in how he processes information. The following quote is used with his permission:

> "I guess I was always somewhat dyslexic, but I didn't know it until I was an adult. When I was a bank teller, I was very close to being fired because I could never balance the accounts at the end of the night. It was usually because of a transposition of a number. I really noticed it later when I started working in jobs where you're always on the phone and people give you phone numbers. I'll hear all the numbers, but I don't conceive an order. I know the numbers are all there, and I can reproduce all the numbers back to you, but I don't even have a best guess of what order they came in if I hear them quickly. That's only true with things like phone numbers because they don't have a natural order that you can re-sort.

> "But there [are] some offsetting advantages to this difficulty, it turns out, for creative types of things. For one, I'm an incredible Scrabble® player because when I look at the letters, they're dancing back and forth on their own, so I don't have to play very hard.

"But there's a correlation to dyslexia and creativity. When I look at things, they don't have to look right to me. I'm comfortable with things looking wrong. I've often defined creativity as the ability to do something wrong and art as the ability to know which ones to keep.

"With Dilbert, for example, he doesn't have a mouth. If Dilbert were designed by a committee he'd have one, because the committee would know that people have mouths. They'd have lots of good reasons. If we're going to animate someday, he'd have to have a mouth because that's where your emotion is. And not only that, he has no eyeballs! The whole value of a cartoon character is that they've got emotion and they show that with their eyes and their mouths! If you don't have one, you've got to have the other! Why didn't I include them? Truth is, I don't know why. It's simply wrong and I choose to keep it that way because it doesn't bother me. There's something total that makes him right, that makes him better because of all these defects. If you designed it right it would just be wrong." (Adams 1996)

2. *Albert Einstein on visual thinking*

Einstein reported he was led to his discoveries by asking questions that only children ask and because his basic thinking was performed without language. He felt his intellectual development was retarded and stated, "as a result of which I began to wonder about space and time only when I had already grown up. Naturally I could go deeper into the problem than a child with normal abilities." (Einstein to James Frank, West 1997, 25)

"The words or the language, as they are spoken or written, do not seem to play any role in my mechanism of thought. The psychical entities which seem to serve as elements in thought are certain signs and more or less clear images which can be "voluntarily" reproduced and combined . . . . These elements are, in my case, of visual and some of muscular type. Conventional words or other signs have to be sought for laboriously only in a second stage when the mentioned associative play is sufficiently established and can be reproduced at will." (West, 26)

3. *Eileen Simpson, Ph.D., novelist, on vocabulary, reading, and good days/bad days*

Eileen describes frequent difficulties with slips of the tongue; for example, saying, "The birds are losing their leaves" (rather than feathers).

> "If, when I made a slip of the tongue, I put on a droll expression or if, when I made an awkward gesture, I gave it a Chaplin-esque flourish, my audience sees mocking and began applauding. This act was not easy to bring off. It required alertness as well as timing and practice. Above all, it was essential to suppress the sense of shock I felt at each fresh bit of evidence that my skull housed an unruly brain." (Simpson 1979, 59)

Many children often have trouble keeping their places while reading. A tendency to skip lines when reading can be misinterpreted as visual acuity problems or, even worse, as an indication that the child is fooling around and not paying attention.

> "The day Miss Henderson observed that I skipped whole lines as well as words when I read, she sent me home with a note suggesting that my vision be checked. Auntie and I set off for the optometrist's office in high spirits, hoping for a cure . . . The optometrist dashed our hopes: vision—20/20." (Simpson 1979, 28)

Eileen further discusses the ongoing symptoms of dyslexia, explaining some of the many inconsistencies, and the resultant frustrations.

> "Since there is no cure for dyslexia, when I say that I was willing to think of myself as 'cured,' what I mean is not that I was or am symptom-free but that my symptoms are manageable—at least on good days. On good days I spell reasonably well . . . Spelling remains hard work—such hard work that I am an untrusty proofreader of my own copy. (Simpson 1979, 217)

> "I have never learned to read and eat at the same time, as during a solitary meal I've wished I could do. Nor can I attend to two competing sounds—a voice and a radio, two people talking to me simultaneously—even on good days.

> "On bad days, which are brought upon by fatigue, preoccupations, illness . . . I have little confidence in my ability to spell . . . . Numbers become scrambled so that I misdial, misaddress, and miscalculate three-quarters of the time. In conversation I might say that Columbus discovered America in 1942 and wonder why people are amused." (Simpson 1979, 218-219)

4. Nelson A. Rockefeller (1908-1979), Vice-President of the United States, 1974-1977, on reading aloud

Rockefeller talks about his dyslexia and the humiliation he suffered as a child because he could not read out loud. He says that even as an adult reading out loud was so difficult for him that he had to have long words in his text broken into syllables and sentences broken into segments. Then, experienced as he was, he "may have to rehearse it six times." (Simpson, 239)

After watching a program on learning disabled children called *The Puzzle Children*, this public figure wrote the following which was published in *T.V. Guide* magazine:

> "I was one of the puzzled children myself, a dyslexic or reverse reader, and I still have a hard time reading today. But after coping with this problem for more than 60 years, I have a message of encouragement for children with learning disabilities . . . . Don't accept anyone's verdict that you are lazy, stupid, or retarded. You may very well be smarter than most other children your age. You can learn to cope with your problem . . . Face the challenge . . . Never quit." (Rockefeller, 1976)

5. Dwayne on creative coping skills

Dyslexics tend to develop very significant coping skills to avoid detection and the subsequent humiliation and frustrations. The situation of filling out a job application, because of its importance, provides one example of the necessity of good coping skills. When Dwayne was handed an application to fill out, he became creative.

He suddenly looked at his watch and said, "I didn't realize it was so late. I have a doctor's appointment. May I bring this back tomorrow?" or "My father's circling the block in all this traffic. Suppose I take this home and return it later?" Then at home his mother would fill out the application and give it to him to return. (Smith 1968, 9)

6. Sir Winston Churchill, Prime Minister of Great Britain, 1940-45 and 1951-55, on superior memory skills

Winston Churchill had great difficulty in school and he was at the bottom of his class. However, he used his superior memory skills as a significant compensation. It was generally known that Churchill had an unusually good memory. However, it is not often point-ed out that Churchill's classmates and masters found his capacity for memo-rization to be "surprising for a student who appeared to be so weak in nearly all other areas." (West 1997, 151)

> "It is thought incongruous that while I apparently stagnated in the lowest form, I should gain a prize open to the whole school for recit-ing to the headmaster 1200 lines of Macaulay's *Lays of Ancient Rome* without making a single mistake." (Churchill 1930, 16-18)

Churchill was very easily distracted and when dictating his speeches or his books, he needed absolute quiet.

> "Any noise, especially high-pitched, was an abomination, especially the jangling of cow bells or whistling, and he lost his train of thought. This extreme sensitivity to noise and difficulty relegating background noise to the background is likely part of the reason for Churchill's unusual working hours, reportedly 11 p.m. until 3 or 4 a.m." (West 1997, 154)

7. *Louise Clarke, author, describing the reading process*
Louise began investigating reading problems in her efforts to understand the school problems her very bright son was experiencing. As she learned about dyslexia, she became aware of her own dyslexic characteristics.

> "I've since analyzed the manner in which words are imprinted on my memory, and there is a definite pattern in the twist the symbols take. Words either follow this pattern or become hopelessly jum-bled. Ordinarily I tend to speak or read the first two letters cor-rectly. Then I skip to the third syllable, which registers either forward or backward; I come back to the second and finish. One of the simpler examples is lethargy, which is 'lagarthy' to me. Other examples are 'dieturic' (diuretic) and 'deddragation' (degradation)." (Clarke 1973, 98)

Summary on vignettes

One of the commonalities among these successful personalities is that they all experienced significant inconsistencies in their performances. The extent of the inconsistencies can be very perplexing within any learning disability.

A student may learn to spell a word but then not be able to maintain that spelling while thinking of other aspects. This tendency to distraction is especially evident during tests. In the example in Figure 4.3 on page 59, Eli, as a second grader,

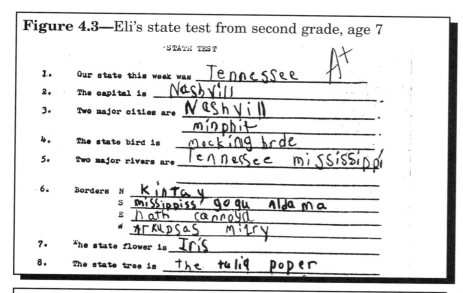

Figure 4.3—Eli's state test from second grade, age 7

STATE TEST

1. Our state this week was *Tennessee* A+
2. The capital is *Nashvill*
3. Two major cities are *Nashvill minphit*
4. The state bird is *mocking brde*
5. Two major rivers are *Tennessee mississippi*
6. Borders N *Kintay*
   S *mississ gogu Aldama*
   E *nath cannoya*
   W *Arkupsas Miry*
7. The state flower is *Iris*
8. The state tree is *the tuliq poper*

Figure 4.4—Eli's E-mail sent from college at age 20

```
MOM & DAD...I used ralphs gift certificat to
get some fud and thank you for the pizza it
was verrrry good...I have never had that kind
befor it tatsed pritty good...we did get to
go to diskneland tho cuz the lectrikul prade
was held off to nov 1st...

This message sent to dad and mom both...to
inshure it benig red!!
```

learned how to spell *Mississippi* by chanting a rhythm, "Miss-iss-ipp-i." Even so, on a test his spelling is inconsistent. He misspelled it once and wrote it correctly another time. Among the other misspellings in this sample are *Kentucky* ("Kintay") and *Georgia* ("Gogu"), which indicate substantial phonological awareness difficulties. Letter reversals are seen in *Alabama* (b/d) and *tulip* (p/q). At age 20, his spelling remains poor (Figure 4.4), especially in situations where he does not use a spell checker, as in this E-mail to his parents.

Explaining and Experiencing Some of the Processing Difficulties to Others

The following simulations are provided for you to experience processing difficulties similar to those experienced by some dyslexics. The exercises are also useful as a means of explaining such processing difficulties to others. You'll find the printed exercises on pages 61-62.

After each activity, answer the following questions. These issues form a good starting point for discussions. After you've completed all three simulations, compare and contrast your reactions to each exercise.

1. Did your eyes feel fatigued?
2. Did you feel physical stress; for example, in your forehead?
3. How efficient (and automatic) was your comprehension?
4. How easy or hard was the activity?
5. What were your feelings while performing the activity?

Simulation 1: We read based on patterns

Many students with dyslexia experience difficulty viewing words as an integrated whole. This simulation also demonstrates what happens when tracking eye movement skills are not automatic.

Read this paragraph (page 61) starting at the pointer on the bottom left but do not use your finger or a marker to keep your place; use only your eyes. Read up, moving from bottom to top. For the next line, start at the top and read down, moving from top to bottom. Continue reading up and down until you reach the end.

Simulations 2 and 3: reversals and a poor ability to maintain consistent eye tracking

Reading can be difficult because of substantial reversals and visual difficulty staying on a straight line during the task. When reading the passages on page 62, remember that as adults we are familiar with left/right progression and we have the ability to recognize which letter is which, even if it is only made with a line and a circle (as in b, d, p, q). Students who struggle do not have these skills internalized in an automatic manner. Read each of the following two paragraphs, answering the five questions at the bottom of page 59 after each reading.

Simulation 1

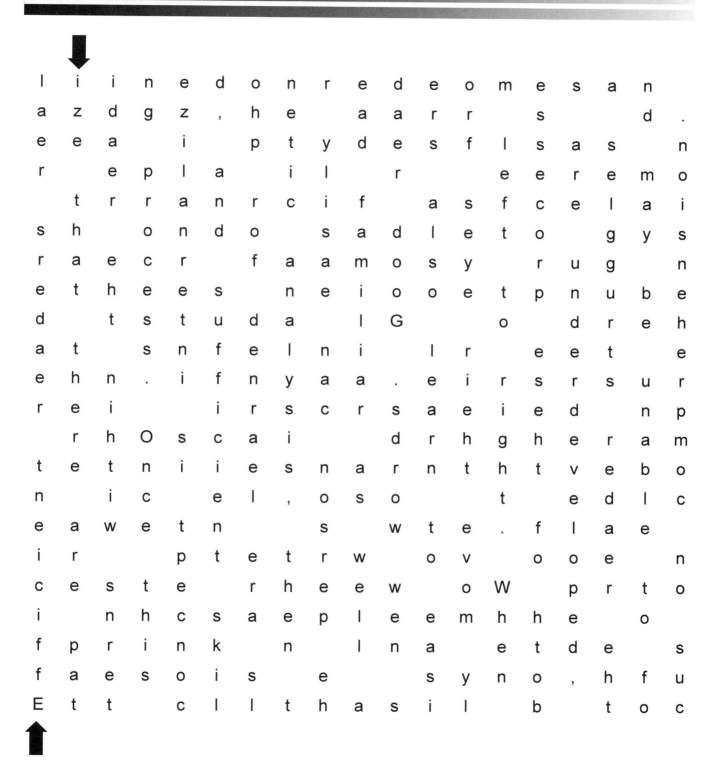

```
l   i   i   n   e   d   o   n   r   e   d   e   o   m   e   s   a   n
a   z   d   g   z   ,   h   e   a   a   r   r   s           d   .
e   e   a       i   p   t   y   d   e   s   f   l   s   a   s       n
r       e   p   l   a       i   l       r       e   e   r   e   m   o
    t   r   r   a   n   r   c   i   f       a   s   f   c   e   l   a   i
s   h       o   n   d   o       s   a   d   l   e   t   o       g   y   s
r   a   e   c   r       f   a   a   m   o   s   y       r   u   g       n
e   t   h   e   e   s       n   e   i   o   o   e   t   p   n   u   b   e
d       t   s   t   u   d   a       l   G           o       d   r   e   h
a       t   s   n   f   e   l   n   i       l   r       e   e   t       e
e   h   n   .   i   f   n   y   a   a   .   e   i   r   s   r   s   u   r
r   e   i       i   r   s   c   r   s   a   e   i   e   d       n   p
    r   h   O   s   c   a   i           d   r   h   g   h   e   r   a   m
t   e   t   n   i   i   e   s   n   a   r   n   t   h   t   v   e   b   o
n       i   c       e   l   ,   o   s   o           t       e   d   l   c
e   a   w   e   t   n           s       w   t   e   .   f   l   a   e
i   r           p   t   e   t   r   w       o   v       o   o   e       n
c   e   s   t   e       r   h   e   e   w       o   W       p   r   t   o
i       n   h   c   s   a   e   p   l   e   e   m   h   h   e       o
f   p   r   i   n   k       n       l   n   a       e   t   d   e       s
f   a   e   s   o   i   s       e       s   y   n   o   ,   h   f   u
E   t   t       c   l   l   t   h   a   s   i   l       b       t   o   c
```

Simulation 2

An old wom an dakeb some gin gerdreab. She hab some bough left ov er, so she mabe the sha be of a little man. She mape eyes, anoseand a smil ing mouth andpl aceq curra ntsbown his front to look like du ttons. Thenshe laib hi mon a qak ingtray and put himint he oven. After a while, som ething rattlebat theo ven boor. She ope nedit and out ju mped the littlegin gerdreab man. She triep to catch him duthes lippeb dast her, ca llingas he ran, "Run, run, as fast as you can. You can't catch me, I'm the gingerdreab man!"

Simulation 3

The$_r$ewa sa sto^{ry} ^{bou}t theth r$_e$ ^{d}$_{ill}$y $^b{_o}^at{_s}$ bru^{ff}. The^r ewa $_s$a ^{gi}b $^d{_i}$ll ydo at' a m$_i$b$_b$l esiz$_e{_b}$ gi^{ll} yg^o$_a$t ' an b a $_l$^{ttl}e o e. $_{Th}^{e}_s$ eth^r^{e}e $^d{_i}$ll^y d^{o}at swa$_n{_t}$^{e}d ni$_{ce}$ br^{en} d^r^{as}s, ^{b}ut they had t$_o$ wal^k^{a}^{n}c$_r$os$_s$ a $_{dri}$^{b}ge t$_o$ g$_e$t $^t{_o}$ $_t$he ne$_w$ t^a ll dr$_a$s^s o^n t$_h$e ot$_h$ er s$_i$de. Bu^t t$_h$e^y ha^b a pr$_o$ble$_m$. Un$_{de}$r the g^{r}ib$_{ge}$ li^v$_e$d a bi$_{dt}$ro l$_l$.

Chapter 5

Symptoms of Dysgraphia

Many students are unfairly labeled as poorly motivated, careless, lazy, or impulsive. These interpretations may at times be true, but they also may only be what is observed on the surface. In some students there is an underlying reason for use of excessive speed and/or production of messy papers. This could be dysgraphia, a processing pattern which is not within the student's control. An astute teacher or parent may suspect dysgraphic symptoms by observing the student while he is writing.

Specific symptoms which may be noted include:

- Cramped fingers on writing tool
- Odd wrist, body, and paper positions
- Excessive erasures, especially due to faulty letter form
- Inconsistent letter formations and slant
- Irregular letter sizes and shapes
- Unfinished cursive letters
- Inappropriate mixture of upper- and lowercase letters
- Mixture of printed and cursive letters
- Misuse of line and margin
- Poor organization on the page
- Inefficient speed in copying
- Decreased speed of writing
- Excessive speed when writing
- General illegibility
- Inattentiveness about details when writing
- Frequent need for verbal cues and use of sub-vocalizing
- Heavy reliance on vision to monitor what the hand is doing during writing

Some students may also demonstrate slow implementation of verbal directions that involve sequencing and planning. While this is not directly involved in the writing process, poor sequencing and planning affect the skills related to writing.

Dysgraphia Is a Problem with the Writing Process

Dysgraphia is primarily a processing problem, that is, an impairment in the process of writing rather than merely a poor product or end result. It affects how the student performs. Looking at a student's written result does not necessarily determine if he is dysgraphic. Similar-looking products (i.e., written results) may be produced by a student with delayed skills (those that are slower in developing), poor writing habits, or dysgraphia (a scatter or disorganization in the processes involved). The student with delayed skills processes adequately, but the product, the designs copied or letters written, may be at a level common to a lower developmental age. The same form orientation, sequence of movement, and timing would all be considered adequate in a younger student. The child with the delay is merely slow to develop copying and writing skills, but does not have a major problem in the ability to retrieve, plan, and make rapid changes in motor movements.

When compared to the child with a delay, the child with poor processing may generate similar-looking letters, especially where the letters are considered individually. However, the way in which this child sequences the movements while writing and the child's timing or fluency are generally inconsistent and/or impaired. These students have significant difficulty with reciprocity, the ability to utilize automatic serial motor movements, such as those required for letter forms. They struggle greatly, exerting excessive effort. Sometimes their written letters actually may look accurate because they use visual analysis to guide their movements.

With enough effort and time, a dysgraphic student may produce an adequate-looking and sometimes neat paper. However, because such a student has weak motor memory, he may form a letter several different ways within the same sentence; the weak motor memory interferes with being able to retrieve a consistent motor plan to form the letter or number. Consequently, he thinks about the formation almost each time, resulting in a cognitive (not automatic) performance that is inconsistent and may contain many erasures. Only by watching the writing process will an astute teacher or parent observe that the child forms the same letter using different sequences throughout the sample, or that the child needs to think about how to create specific letters. Some students appear as though they are drawing each letter. Sometimes the student may actually stop and ask how to form a given letter.

There are many degrees of dysgraphia. Some children can trace within boundaries and are able to copy or draw a simple design. However, they are unable to develop automatic consistencies for forming letters. They struggle to copy figures that require reciprocal movements and contain a repetitive pattern. Some students, especially those who are older and have practiced writing a great deal, can

Figure 5.1a—drawing by a 12-year-old dysgraphic student: "A Castle in Zeal"

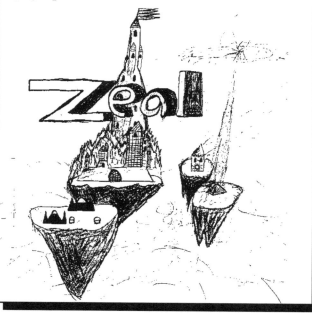

Figure 5.2a—"Megaman," a drawing by a 10-year-old dysgraphic student

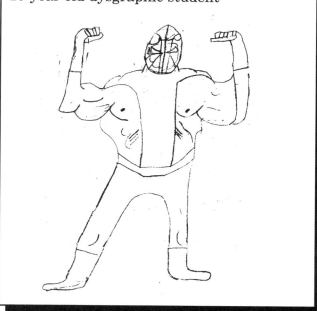

Figure 5.1b—dysgraphic writing sample by same 12-year-old

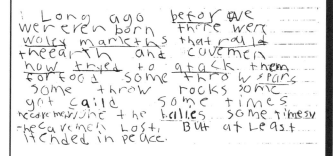

Translation:

Long ago, before we were even born there were wooly mammoths that ruled the earth and cavemen who tried to attack them for food some threw (throw) spears some threw (throw) rocks some got killed sometimes the cavemen won (one) the battles (balies) sometimes the cavemen lost. But at least it ended in peace.

Figure 5.2b—dysgraphic writing sample by same 10-year-old

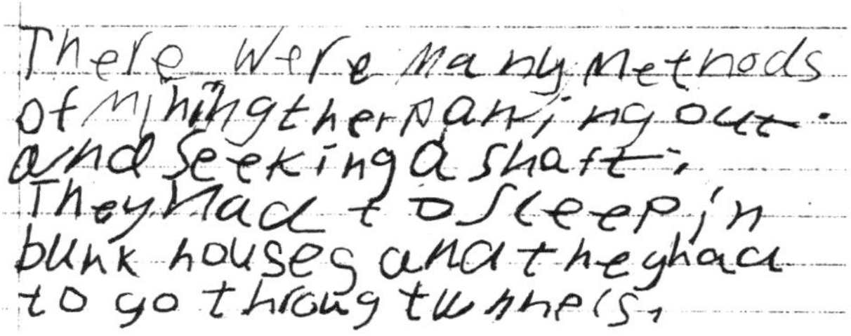

Translation:

There were many methods of mining their panning out and seeking a shaft. They had to sleep in bunk houses and they had to go through tunnels.

sometimes produce legible writing; however, closer observation of their techniques indicates distorted sequences of movements. These students visually know what the letters and the words look like, but do not automatically recall the proper motoric movements to create those images.

Adults are often perplexed by artistic children who struggle greatly with the task of writing. This can be a disadvantage for these children who may then be accused of not caring about the writing. When the motor function is liberated from sequential memory, such children can demonstrate a strong fine motor performance, which results in artistic creative drawings. The figures on page 65 provide examples of artistic dysgraphic students.

Many of these artistic students have described the process of writing as being similar to drawing. Such a student states that he has a visual image of the letters in his head, and he matches his motor movements to that visual image. This then becomes a *visual* process rather than an *automatic motor movement* process. These children tend to have excellent capabilities for imaging and visualizing objects, space, and form, and they are able to translate these images into a visual representation with varying degrees of ease and efficiency. However, the process of writing letters or numbers requires a *sequential motor memory* to enable students to remember the sequences of lines and circles required for individual letters.

This process of forming letters is very different from recreating or drawing objects such as flowers, cars, or animals. In dysgraphia, the sequential motor memory difficulties create the struggles with letters and numbers and interfere with automaticity. An analogy can be made with the dyslexic student who displays good verbal fluency when he is in charge of the topic. However, when asked a direct question or required to conform to a structure, he may struggle greatly to remember words and organize his thoughts.

Difficulty with motor memory is one of the most common causes of handwriting difficulty and a major contributor to dysgraphia. (Levine 1987, 208-239) For motor sequences such as letter formations to become automatic, the motor patterns must be firmly established and rapidly recalled, with very little conscious thought. In contrast, dysgraphic students need to consciously remember how to form certain letters, resulting in hesitation; poor, unsteady rhythm; and lack of smoothness in form. Sometimes they may produce a letter and immediately recognize it as incorrect. They cross out, erase, or retrace letters in their attempts to maximize the correctness of the visual product. Sometimes they seem surprised by the production of a wrong letter, as though the correct letter was requested but the wrong letter was sent out to be produced by the hand. Parents and teachers are often puzzled by the difficulties these children experience with writing, especially if the same children demonstrate good athletic skills and fine motor abilities when drawing. Drawing and most other motor skills do not demand as much recall of precise, automatic, sequential motor patterns. Instead they rely on movements that involve more visual guidance and decision-making as they are performed.

There are six possible factors that exacerbate motor memory problems. The first two factors almost always indicate dysgraphia and the last two factors by themselves rarely indicate dysgraphia.

- Weak kinesthetic memory so that an accurate pattern is not stored
- Poor ability to express written ideas with clarity and in sequence, especially when the student is more efficient when verbally expressing clear, sequential ideas
- Generalized memory or sequencing weakness
- Weak or inconsistent ability to recall visual and motoric movement sequences
- Inexperience due to lack of practice involving consistent repetition of the pattern
- Lack of experience due to attentional problems

The Motor Plan

The major handwriting problem for dysgraphic students is difficulty formulating or implementing the motor plan, especially as reciprocity (the ability to change directions adequately and fluently) is required. Variability exists among these students. Some may not form a good mental image of what they intend to write (such as the letter form) and some may produce an adequate mental image but cannot execute it. Both aspects result in a slow written output, with noticeable lack of automaticity in forming letters and spacing words. Figure 5.3 demonstrates an example of manuscript writing by a student who has great difficulty with letter form.

For some students, the memory storage for a cursive word is one long serial chain. This requires more complex

---

Figure 5.3—A story written to match a picture prompt by a very bright student age 8-5. Note difficulties with spacing and consistency.

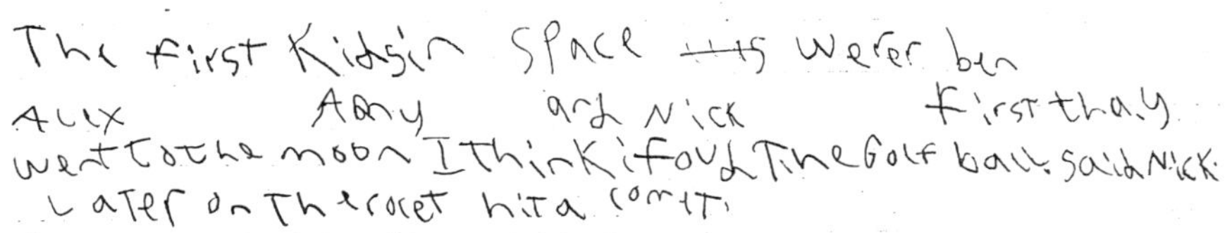

Translation:
The first kids in space were Ben, Alex, Amy, and Nick. First they went to the moon. I think I found the golf ball, said Nick. Later on the rocket hit a comet. [Note: Last names were omitted.]

---

motor sequences, making the production of words and sentences more difficult. In contrast, printing provides opportunities for breathers since each letter is formed separately from the others and is recalled as a separate, short movement sequence.

Thus, for some dysgraphics, printing facilitates memory storage and retrieval and is often the preferred writing mode. However, with sufficient and appropriate practice, these students can and do learn to write in cursive, although this mode may remain slow and/or laborious.

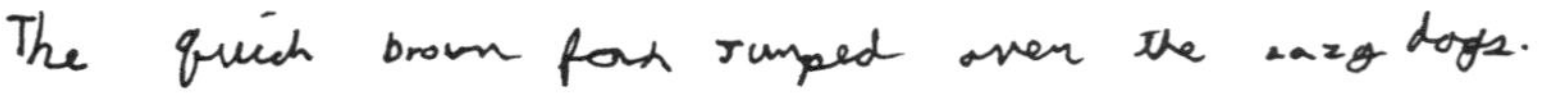

At age 21, Eli (from Chapter 1) was asked to copy the sentence "The quick brown fox jumped over the lazy dogs." He was asked to use cursive and write as fast as he could. He copied the sentence twice. (Figures 5.4a

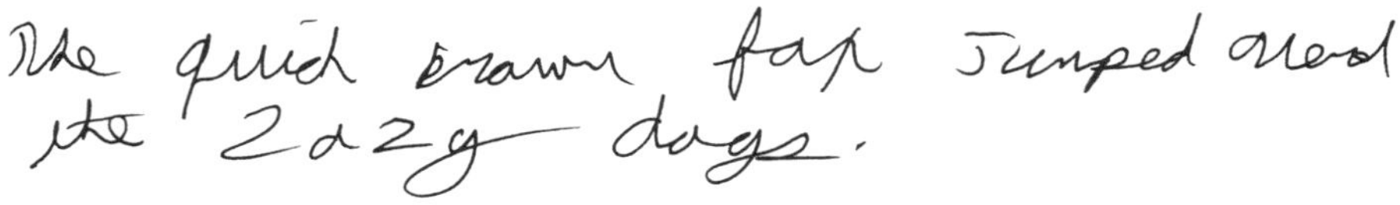

Sentences copied by Eli at age 21.

Figure 5.4a

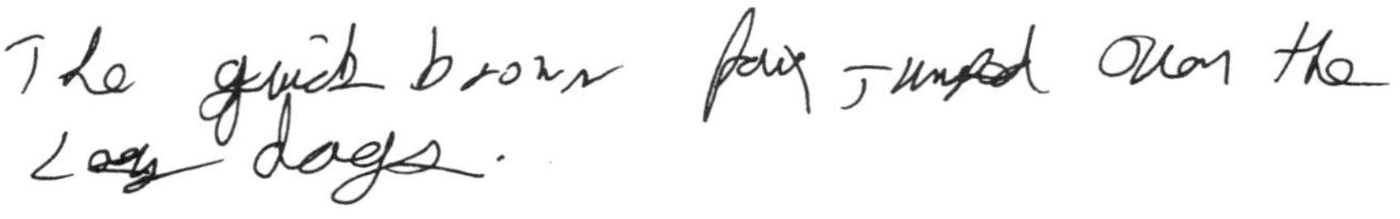

The quick brown fox jumped over the lazy dogs.

Figure 5.4b

The quick brown fox jumped over the lazy dogs.

Figure 5.4c

The quick brown fox jumped over the lazy dogs.

and 5.4b) He was then asked to copy it again making it as neat and clear as possible. Without direct awareness, he automatically decreased the size of his letters in his attempt to achieve more control. (Figure 5.4c) Although he is able to write in cursive, he prefers manuscript.

Many children with weak motor memory have above average visual perception and analysis skills. They may depend greatly on visual comparison and correction because they cannot depend on their motor recall for accurate letter and number formation. In other words, they need to see what they write before determining its correctness. Some children, however, struggle with this aspect of visual imagery and visual comparisons. These children may not recognize a form when its size is changed or when details are added, and may have difficulty reading different type styles or changing from manuscript to cursive writing.

Inconsistencies

Written expression skills among dysgraphic children vary considerably. Some do not discriminate the difference between upper- and lowercase letters when writing paragraphs. Many make substantial mechanical errors in spelling, grammar, and punctuation because of the interrelationship of writing within the complete language cluster. Sometimes these children can explain complex ideas verbally but cannot write at a similar level of complexity.

A major contributor to this particular aspect of the problem is that these students often have a reduced active working memory, a recall aspect enabling them to hold components in mind while working on parts of the task. Efficiency with active working memory enables the learner to return to an earlier step in a task and process and integrate it with other elements. We can envision active working memory as a screen (such as that on a television monitor or the menu page on a computer) on which data are stored while in use. The screen needs to be clear enough and large enough so that all components of the task are readily available while at the same time leaving enough space to work on the task.

When students enter upper elementary grades, a greater degree of automization is required. They are expected to produce an increased volume of writing while sustaining attention to detail and self-monitoring. Active working memory becomes essential. A student must simultaneously maintain the meaning of a sentence while trying to find the right vocabulary and remembering to capitalize, punctuate, and spell correctly. At this stage of development, it is often common for students to lose track of their thought processes and forget what they are writing. Developmentally most students progress beyond this difficulty, but students with dysgraphia become stuck in this developmental problem. So much of their cognitive energy is spent at the mechanical level (which should be automatic!) that the capacity of their active working memory becomes greatly reduced.

Figure 5.5—Summarization of a paragraph heard aurally, written by 10th grade student with I.Q. score in gifted range.

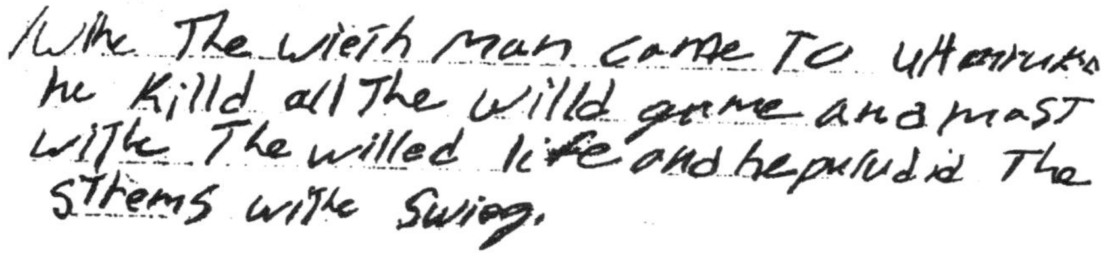

Translation:
When (Wihe) the white man came to America (uhmruka) he killed all the wild game and messed with the wild life and he polluted the streams with sewage.

Figures 5.5, 5.6, and 5.7 present writing samples by students who scored in the gifted range on an I.Q. test. These students performed with excellent accuracy when given lists of sentences to capitalize or punctuate. In Figure 5.5, a 15-year-old wrote a summary of a short passage that was read to him. This increases the demands placed on his active working memory because he must retain the paragraph in mind while also organizing and remembering what he wants to write. Figure 5.6 presents a story the same student wrote to correspond to a picture prompt. In this situation, the prompt remains in front of him, reducing the need for him to retain the picture in his own mind. Figure 5.7 on page 71 presents a story by a nine-year-old student who thrives on being creative.

Figure 5.6—Story written in response to a picture prompt from *Test of Written Language* (TOWL-3). Same 10th grade student as Figure 5.5.

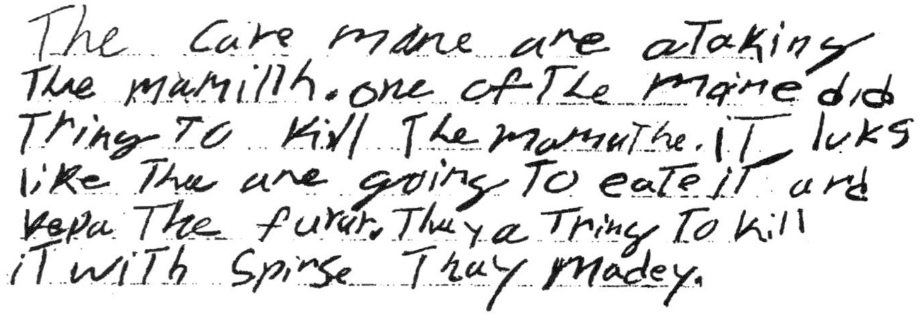

Translation:
The cavemen are attacking the mammoth. One of the men died trying to kill the mammoth. It looks like they are going to eat it and keep the fur. They are trying to kill it with spears they made.

As students mature, they are expected to consolidate a greater range of information into larger amounts of writing, a process demanding sustained, selective attention; self-monitoring; and the maintenance of priorities in active working memory. Reduced active working memory and the need to process a range of information causes *processing fatigue*. The automatic writing of letters is an integration of many component parts and the dysfluency of these foundational components contributes to lack of endurance. This, plus a motor weakness resulting in poor automatization of the motor movements required for writing causes a *motor fatigue*. There is a critical interaction between motor fatigue and processing fatigue. This is what Levine refers to as a dysfunction of the junction between the functions. (Levine 1993) The degree of overall fatigue varies greatly within each individual and with each task. This causes substantial *inconsistency*, which is one of the most perplexing and least understood aspects of dysgraphia. Figure 5.8 on page 72 presents samples from a 10-year-old. Note the large and inconsistent letter form and his switch from cursive to manuscript for different tasks.

With sufficient time and motivation, the student with dysgraphia will occasionally produce an exemplary paper. A child may work hard and produce a neat line of print, but the paper may be neat for only the first line or two. As the task progresses, the student's efficiency decreases. This intermittent success leads parents and teachers to falsely believe the unacceptable work is the result of laziness or carelessness.

It is true that handwriting improves with practice, but there is a time/energy ratio that is crucial in understanding the dysgraphic student's ability to produce an occasionally satisfactory written product. A dysgraphic student often develops

Figure 5.7—Story by a very bright nine-year-old student in response to a picture prompt from the *Test of Written Language* (TOWL-3). Her inconsistencies in pencil pressure are quite noticeable.

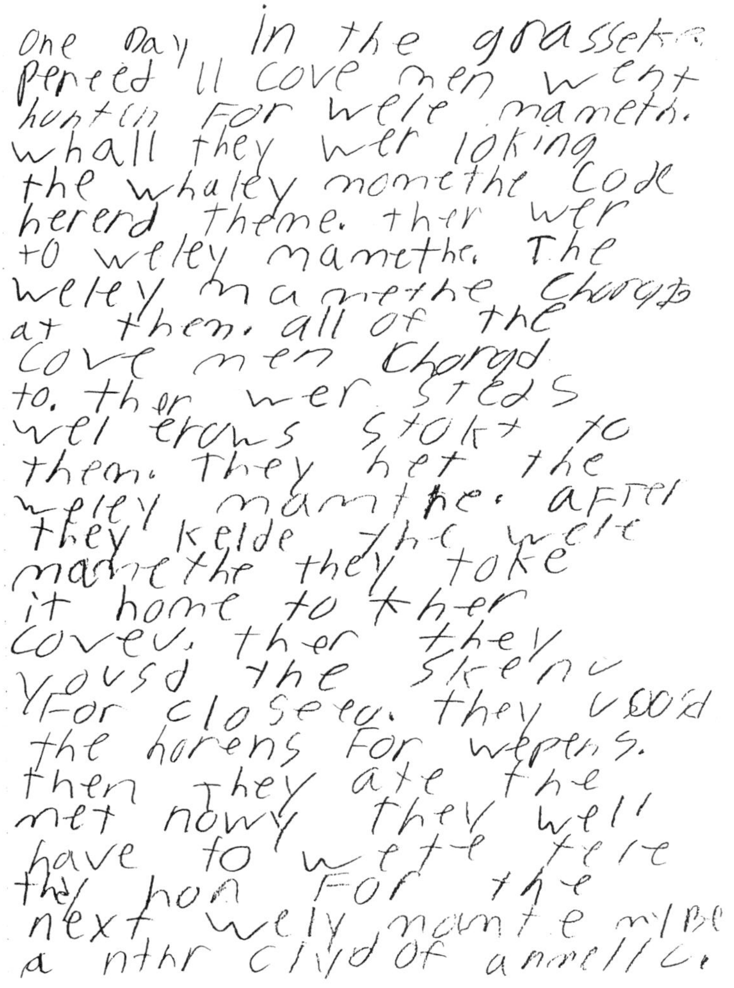
One Day in the grassekr
pereed 11 cove men went
huntin For wele maneth.
whall they wer loking
the whaley momethe Code
herend theme. ther wer
to weley manethe. The
weley manethe Chorgd
at them. all of the
cove men Chorgd
to. ther wer steds
wel erows stokt to
them. They het the
weley mamthe. aFTel
they kelde the wele
manethe they toke
it home to ther
cove. ther they
yousd the skene
For closeeu. they useed
the horens For wepens.
then they ate the
met nowy they well
have to wete tere
they hon For the
next wely mamte mlBe
a nthr clyd of anmells.

Translation:
One day in the Jurassic period 11 cavemen went hunt for wooly mammoths. While they were looking the wooly mammoth could hear them. There were two wooly mammoth. The woooley mammoths charged at them. All of the cavemen charged too. There were sticks with arrows stuck to them. They hit the wooly mammoth. After they killed the wooly mammoth they took it home to their cave. There they used the skin for clothes. They used the horns for weapons. Then they ate the meat. Now they will have to wait till they hunt for the next wooly mammoth maybe another kind of animals.

many compensations to deal with the particular aspects of writing that cause difficulty. While these may help with a single aspect, it is generally difficult to integrate a variety of compensations simultaneously. Furthermore, excessive use of compensations generally leads to excessive fatigue; inefficient energy expenditure; and slow, poor formation of letters. The length and complexity of a given writing task contribute to the degree to which such symptoms appear. Longer and more complex tasks cause skills to become more unreliable and decrease endurance, thereby resulting in overall task inefficiency.

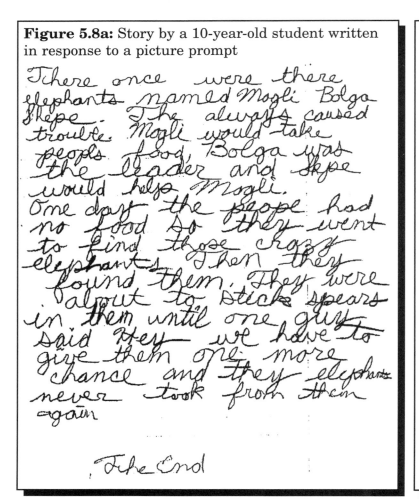

Figure 5.8a: Story by a 10-year-old student written in response to a picture prompt

Figure 5.8b: Dictated, unpracticed spelling test written by the same student

Understanding Dysgraphia: A Summary

Dysgraphia is defined as "a writing pattern characterized by substantial effort which interferes with a student's ability to convert ideas into a written format." The basic prerequisite skills for letter form and use of space are inefficient, causing great energy drain and consequently interfering with the higher level performances of expression using a written format. Primarily, the student experiences difficulty in automatically remembering and mastering the sequence of muscle motor movements needed in writing letters or numbers. It is a difficulty which is out of harmony with the person's intelligence, regular teaching instruction, and (in most cases) the use of the pencil in non-learning tasks. It is an unexpected underachievement—an unexpected underachievement based on the student's strong skills in other areas.

Dysgraphia . . .

- is a processing problem
- causes writing fatigue
- interferes with communication of ideas in writing
- contributes to poor organization on the line and on the page

Dysgraphia can be seen in . . .

- letter inconsistencies
- mixture of upper/lowercase letters or print/cursive letters
- irregular letter sizes and shapes
- unfinished letters
- struggle to use writing as a communications tool

Dysgraphia is not . . .

- laziness
- lack of trying
- lack of caring
- sloppy writing
- general sloppiness
- careless writing
- visual-motor delay

The use of the label *dysgraphia* is not critical, and there may be some situations where the actual label is irrelevant, and its use may even be inappropriate. However, the concept can be useful in generating greater understanding of why some students struggle considerably with the basic mechanics of writing. It is also useful in organizing skill training, especially in younger grades. Recognizing when a writing pattern is not within the range of normal development generates an understanding that the problem may be neurologically based and may exist in varying degrees, ranging from mild to moderate.

Dysgraphia is an inefficiency which seldom exists in isolation or without other symptoms of learning problems. It is most commonly related to learning problems within the sphere of written language and is frequently associated with dyslexia. However, it may also be associated with motor clumsiness or poor spatial awareness. It is one of many developmental problems which affects output or performance. It often results from a variety of different factors, and as such, it affects other tasks which have similar demands or which rely on similar processing mechanisms.

Difficulties with writing often lead to misunderstandings by teachers and parents, and consequently, to many frustrations for the student. This is especially true for the bright, linguistically quick student who encounters a major stumbling block when dealing with written expression, often due to the lack of smooth, efficient automaticity in letter and word formation. These students struggle to translate their thoughts and knowledge, denying their teachers the opportunity to understand what they know.

Dysgraphia can be diagnosed, and it can be overcome if appropriate remedial strategies are taught well and conscientiously carried out. It is important to note, however, that remedial programs generally work more efficiently with younger students because the inefficient habits and patterns are less ingrained. An adequate remedial program works best when applied on a daily basis and reinforced throughout all activities whenever the student uses a pencil. Since this may not be practical in many educational situations, it is effective to also plan appropriate compensations. Compensations or bypass strategies are relatively easy to design once the underlying mechanisms of dysgraphia are more thoroughly understood.

In Chapters 12 and 13 you'll find suggestions for compensations and remediation. While these are particularly critical for the dysgraphic student, the suggestions can also be used efficiently with any student who struggles with writing or avoids writing for other reasons. Remember, the diagnostic label is not what is critical. It is critical, however, to recognize that a student may be having difficulty with writing and then move on to initiate and utilize the appropriate bypass or remedial strategies.

Simulation

Eye/hand coordination can be a struggle for a dysgraphic student; she knows what she wants her hand to do, but her hand does not always cooperate. This simulation allows you to experience similar struggles within a simple drawing activity.

The task is to draw a star, maintaining your lines within the given boundaries. Use a photocopy of the handout on page 76 for this activity. The trick is that you can only look into a mirror. A small mirror on a stand works best.

Hold the mirror perpendicular to the photocopy so that you can see your hand directly in the mirror. Once the mirror is in place, have someone hold a sturdy piece of paper or cardboard between you and the mirror, ideally over your writing hand and below your eyes. Make sure that you can still see your hand and the pencil in the mirror but you cannot directly see what your hand is doing. Adjust the position of the paper or the mirror if necessary. Now look into the mirror and draw the star, maintaining visual awareness on your hand movements within the mirror. While drawing, be sure to keep your line within the boundaries of the star pattern.

Ask your helper to observe these four points so you can discuss them afterwards.

- Are you white-knuckling the pencil?
- If given a comment such as "You're doing well," does it distract your concentration?
- How easily do you shift directions?
- Does your helper notice any signs of frustration or tension in your face?

After you are done, discuss your experience. Then hold the mirror for your helper and repeat the activity.

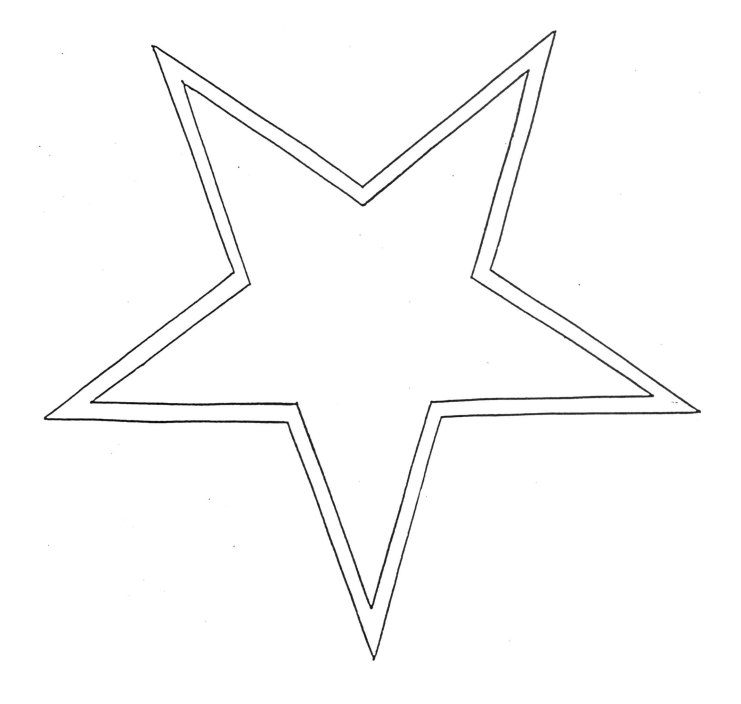

Chapter 6

The Diagnostic Process

The Process of Diagnosing Dyslexia

It is common for many professionals and parents to ask, "What test can I use (or request) to diagnose dyslexia?" The truth is that no single test is sufficient. The diagnostic process is a multidimensional analysis of processing and learning, as recommended by the International Dyslexia Association. (Greene, et al 1995)

Dyslexia cannot be identified by a single number or score on any assessment instrument. As a complex disorder involving language processing, it requires a broad and comprehensive look at many aspects of learning and performance. It is critical for the examiner to analyze the processing used by the student in both oral and written language.

Tests are but a tool in the hands of a knowledgeable evaluator who must recognize what to look for and how to analyze observations and performances. Most available statistically solid assessment tools can be used as a framework, but it is up to the evaluator to structure the situation and use clinical judgement to analyze the nature of responses and compare the child's performances with expectancies. The key to successful diagnoses of any processing disorder involves the efficiency of the examiner's analytical skills.

Three areas must be assessed to consider a diagnosis of dyslexia: cognitive ability; skills in language, reading, and

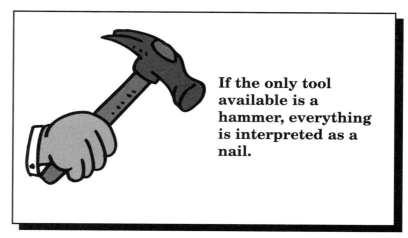

If the only tool available is a hammer, everything is interpreted as a nail.

writing; and processing components. School psychologists, educational psychologists, and sometimes clinical psychologists are skilled in assessing cognition and academics. Special educators and speech and language pathologists efficiently test reading, writing, and language skills. However, when considering processing components, the examiner's degree obtained (whether a doctorate or a master's level) is not as important as the training, philosophy, and experience of the examiner. There are many fine professionals with masters' degrees who are quite skilled in assessing the processing involved in language, reading, and writing. Learning to thoroughly and accurately analyze a student's processing requires substantial study and experience and an ability to use a test as a tool rather than merely to generate numbers.

Many researchers and writers have described the process of diagnosing dyslexia. (Clark 1995, Cramer 1996, Greene 1995, Hall & Moats 1999, Levine 1998, Lyon 1994, West 1997) The following is the process I use, as developed and modified through more than two decades of involvement with the International Dyslexia Association, intensive study, and private practice experience. Tests in the cognitive domain and many of the language areas need to be administered by professionals with the appropriate license or credential (psychologist and speech/language pathologist). The remaining educational areas may be assessed and analyzed by a trained educator with an appropriately related degree and/or credential. Keep in mind that the goal is description of the student, not generation of scores.

Components Relevant to the Diagnostic Process to Determine Dyslexia

Diagnostic Area	Components included
Family and individual history	✔ Relatives who have had or are having difficulties in reading, writing, and spelling ✔ Health or medical impairments to learning, including early history of ear infections ✔ Delays in beginning to speak and/or history of unusual word pronunciations ✔ Parents' concerns regarding speech, language, motor skills, attentional issues, and academics ✔ Parents' goals for the assessment

Diagnostic Area	Components included
Cognitive ability and intellectual aptitude	✔ Assessment of strengths and weaknesses in cognitive skills ✔ Individual's aptitude for learning in a variety of areas ✔ Identification that student has average or above average cognitive potential
Specific language skills	✔ Speech sound and syllable awareness/manipulation skills ✔ Word pronunciation/sound articulation ✔ Word retrieval and rapid automatic naming ✔ Rhyming skills ✔ Knowledge of word meanings and ability to define words ✔ Comprehension and production of sentence structure (syntax and morphology) ✔ Comprehension of what is heard ✔ Expressive ability, including organization of ideas, elaboration, and clarity of expression ✔ Expressive ability to summarize a paragraph heard ✔ Expressive ability to formulate questions
Single-word decoding (word accuracy)	✔ Individual sound/symbol correspondence (especially with young students) ✔ Accurate reading of single words presented in a list (i.e., no context) ✔ Use of word attack skills when reading nonsense words ✔ Oral reading fluency and accuracy, especially of paragraphs (i.e., within context)
Reading comprehension	✔ Timed reading of longer passages read silently ✔ Comprehension of material read silently ✔ Comprehension of material read orally ✔ Use of context clues and logical reasoning to determine meaning when many words are misread or unknown ✔ Comparison of factual and inferential comprehension skills

Diagnostic Area	Components included
Spelling	✔ Use of invented spelling (especially with young students) ✔ Dictated written spelling test, to include analysis of errors—sound additions or omissions, confusion of letter sequences, poor memory for common patterns ✔ Multiple choice spelling test (to determine ease of using spell checker and to compare with written spelling performance) ✔ Written composition (story or essay) to analyze use of spelling within context
Written expression	✔ Sentence writing ✔ Story writing to analyze word choice; quality and complexity of sentences, ideas, and grammar; use of punctuation and capitalization ✔ Tasks such as writing a paraphrase, combining simple sentences into compound and complex sentences, writing an outline, writing part of a structured paragraph, writing a topic sentence ✔ Comparison of use of skills in isolation and in contextual writing
Handwriting	✔ Ability to form letters alone and in words ✔ Analysis of use of space, lines, letter form, letter slant ✔ Analysis of consistency and slant ✔ Hand used for writing and pencil grip used ✔ Positioning of hand and rotation of paper
Memory	✔ Episodic memory (often through parent and/or self reports) ✔ Long-term memory (general information, vocabulary) ✔ Rote sequential memory (months of year, days of week, math facts) ✔ Visual memory for details, form, and sequences (often a strength is identified which can be used in remediation) ✔ Comparison of auditory and visual recall ✔ Analysis of active working memory
Other observations	✔ Rote motor sequences (tying shoes) ✔ Organizational skills ✔ Time management

After assessing and analyzing the information derived from the above areas, the examiner compiles a list of the student's strengths and weaknesses in three areas: 1) oral language, 2) written language (reading and writing), and 3) other. These symptoms and patterns can be compared to the information in Chapter 4, the Symptoms of Dyslexia, to provide a more thorough description of the student. Since dyslexia relates to underlying gaps in language processing, to confirm a dyslexic classification, the following *RET Dyslexia Diagnostic System* can be used wherein the student must demonstrate significant gaps in one or more symptoms in each of the following categories. (*RET Dyslexia Diagnostic System*, 1998)

Dyslexic students exhibit (one or more):	and	Dyslexic students exhibit (one or more):
✗ poor skill and/or significant gaps in phonological awareness ✗ weak automaticity in phonological awareness ✗ reduced rapid automatic naming		✗ poor spelling ✗ reduced spelling in context ✗ slow reading speed and/or fluency ✗ poor language organization and formulation within higher levels of reading comprehension and/or written expression

It is important to note that poor word accuracy (decoding) is not a diagnostic indicator of dyslexia. Although many dyslexics struggle with word accuracy, there are other reasons for poor skill in this area. Additionally, remediated dyslexics may demonstrate accurate decoding skills, but their basic processing gaps continue to affect automaticity and efficiency in one or more areas.

> "An over-reliance on reading has led to intractable practical and theoretical difficulties in the understanding and diagnosis of dyslexia . . . . Even in the well-compensated dyslexic, deficits may still show in the fluency of skills, particularly in reading unfamiliar words, in spelling, in working under time pressure, and in general organizational skills." (Fawcett 1998, 65)

It was common in the early 1990s to consider a reading problem to be a generalized reading problem (also called garden variety) if 1) the student exhibited expressive or receptive language problems in conjunction with reading gaps, or 2) the student's reading performance was similar to his mental ability. (Stanovich 1988, 1991) The proliferation of studies throughout the 1990s has generated a different viewpoint: a dyslexic student may have, and often does have, associated receptive or expressive language difficulties, though sometimes only at the higher, more abstract levels. (Lyon 1997, 23; Vellutino 1997, 36; Hall & Moats 1999, 272, 273, 293)

Identifying and Diagnosing the Dysgraphic Student

Students who struggle to write begin to doubt their skills as a learner. They would benefit if their teachers and/or parents had greater understanding and ability to suspect dysgraphia from the students' sloppy and/or inconsistent writing.

To begin the diagnostic process, it is important to first determine if the writing problem is interfering with learning or the student's ability to demonstrate what he knows. If it is, then the following six areas can be used as guidelines to determine a dysgraphic pattern. Observations within all six areas are required to make a reliable diagnostic statement.

1. **Clusters**

   Use the list of symptoms in the box on the right to identify clusters of symptoms. Look for a pattern. No single symptom indicates dysgraphia.

2. **Feedback and anticipating**

   Observe the student's performance when copying and also when performing spontaneous writing. This is important because each type of writing is dependent upon a different mechanism. Copying requires frequent monitoring of a model, and is, therefore, dependent upon adequate visual feedback. Spontaneous writing requires recall of a motor pattern or engram, and, therefore, is dependent upon anticipating the information processed before the action begins. Many students with dysgraphia have problems with both mechanisms, although some may only struggle with the component involving anticipation.

3. **Rhythm and timing**

   Observe the student's timing and fluency of hand movements. Timing affects the rhythm and flow of writing across the page. Problems with timing can be observed when a student has labored or jerky writing. Rapid, haphazard writing is often the result when a student gives up attempts at controlling movement. Students with timing difficulties struggle to follow a sequential, repetitive series of motor movements in a fluid manner.

4. **Motor difficulties**

   The inability to carry out a sequential motor movement to perform a motor task is often observed in students who

Specific Symptoms which may be noted include:

- ❏ Cramped fingers on writing tool
- ❏ Odd wrist, body, and paper positions
- ❏ Excessive erasures
- ❏ Mixture of upper- and lowercase letters
- ❏ Mixture of printed and cursive letters
- ❏ Inconsistent letter formations and slant
- ❏ Irregular letter sizes and shapes
- ❏ Unfinished cursive letters
- ❏ Misuse of line and margin
- ❏ Poor organization on the page
- ❏ Inefficient speed in copying
- ❏ Decreased speed of writing
- ❏ Excessive speed when writing
- ❏ General illegibility
- ❏ Inattentiveness about details when writing
- ❏ Frequent need for verbal cues and use of sub-vocalizing
- ❏ Heavy reliance on vision to monitor what the hand is doing during writing
- ❏ Slow implementation of verbal directions that involve sequencing and planning

struggle greatly to learn a task such as tying shoes or those who display general clumsiness. These students are awkward in gross motor activities such as running, hopping, or skipping and may have trouble throwing or catching. It is important to note, however, that gross motor clumsiness does not always correlate with dysgraphia. Students with this problem are sometimes labeled as having dysgraphia due to motor clumsiness.

5. Activities requiring reciprocal movements

Difficulty with reciprocity is an important component of a dysgraphic pattern. Consequently, these students struggle with tasks such as copying repetitive designs, as such tasks require reciprocal movements or a fluent changing of directions. Page 86 contains examples of designs for the suspected dysgraphic student to copy. The designs should be drawn, one at a time, large, ideally ten inches high, on a chalkboard. Repeat the form six to eight times. Encourage the child to use the same shape, number of units, and approximate size, saying, "Make yours just like mine." Students may copy underneath the model on the chalkboard or on a large paper, sitting about four feet from the chalkboard and directly in front of the designs. Observe for accuracy of form as well as smooth movements. If a student needs to pause (or stop) at the change of direction, that represents a significant indication of a timing and/or sequencing problem.

Pages 87-89 contain examples of students' performances.

6. Pencil grip

Observe for consistency of grip usage and check the following:

- distance from finger to pencil point (should be consistently between ¾ to 1 inch)
- pressure on pencil (should not be too light or too heavy)
- angle of pencil (should be approximately 45° with page)
- finger control and anchoring of pencil

Page 90 illustrates some common pencil grip positions.

The Written Report

The end result of any assessment should be a complete report presented verbally and in writing to parents, with particular focus on the initial referral questions and goals. A written document is necessary to explain the child to the parents and teachers and may also be needed to substantiate the child's educational status. The report should be thorough and contain much more than a list of test scores. However, the test scores should be fully and completely reported, in a manner that parents can readily comprehend. It is critical that the entire report be in language the parent can understand! The student also needs to be informed of the results, using a format appropriate for her developmental level and including the process of demystification. Levine presents an excellent description of this step:

> "A good prescription should be based on a good description. Once we have compiled and integrated a vivid description of (all) the elements . . . , it becomes possible to share the formulation with the principal actors. We call this process of explication demystification, a process in which a child's plight is described so that it contains as little myth, fantasy, and mystery as possible. Weaknesses and strengths are described in concrete terms . . . and should also serve to convince children and parents of their ability to affect future outcomes." (Levine 1998, 568)

If a diagnostic label of dyslexia or dysgraphia is used, it is important to identify the particular symptoms exhibited by the student. A statement should be included such as, "Eli's dyslexic pattern is substantiated by . . ." This helps avoid semantic misunderstandings and also personalizes the label to the student.

The following sections are recommended as components of a valuable written report, keeping in mind that the purpose of the educational diagnostic evaluation is to clarify and explain the student's profile.

Background

✔ Identifying information regarding the individual

✔ Student's history and background, including any testing performed by other professionals, most importantly as related to cognitive functioning

Summary

✔ Overview summary of student's strengths and weaknesses (may be in graphic format)

✔ Complete summary of strengths and weaknesses in a comprehensive, cohesive explanation (may be included as a summary at end of report)

Interpretations and Observations

✔ Description of observations of student's processing and behaviors, including attention, memory, motor movement, and processing speed

✔ Student's strengths and weaknesses, including test results and processing components

✔ Specific observations regarding the processing components related to each language, academic, and visual area

✔ Interpretive statements regarding each area

Recommendations

✔ Specific recommendations for interventions at home and at school

✔ Recommendations for compensations

✔ Recommendations for remediation

✔ Recommendations for further evaluations, if necessary

It is also beneficial to write the older student a brief letter using language appropriate for his age. The letter should thank the student for his cooperation in the testing process, reinforce his strengths, provide a brief explanation of why he is struggling, and state basic recommendations. The purpose of the letter is to demystify the student's anxiety about any suspicions that he may be stupid, to provide hope that there is help available for him, and to give him some specifics regarding the nature of available assistance. Even if this has been done verbally, it is useful to follow up in writing, as this can become a permanent reminder for the student.

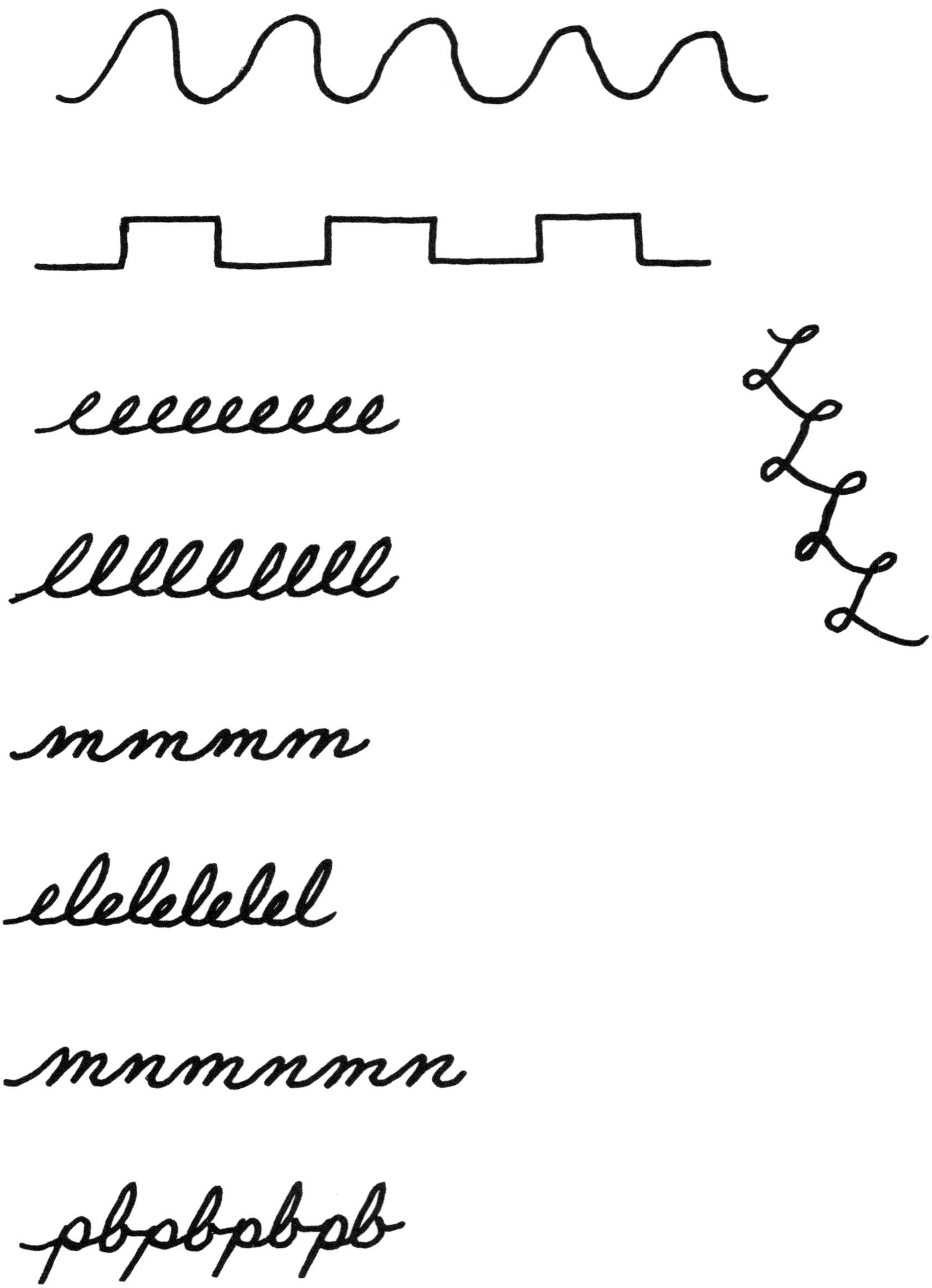

Age 8: Three attempts to copy a tall loop seven times.

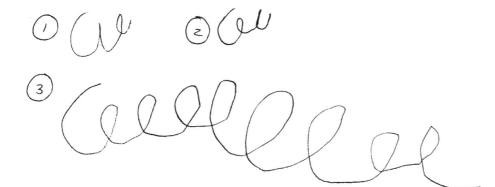

Age 9: Second and third attempts at copying *mn* five times. Notice the great difficulty with shifts—so much that pattern (form) is destroyed.

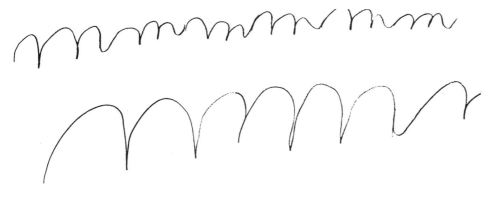

Age 10: Notice retracings, corrections, segmentation, and pattern error on last design.

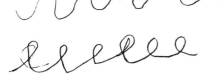

Age 11: This student struggles greatly with reciprocity (directional shifts). First is three sets of *bp;* second is six sets of *le.*

Age 11: This student struggles greatly with reciprocity (directional shifts). In sets of *pb*, notice how he loses the pattern.

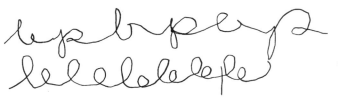

Age 12: Two attempts to copy *bp* four times. Although the form is close to correct, notice segmentation and difficulty with directional shifts on last pattern.

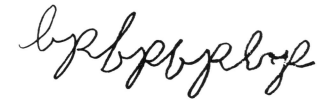

Several attempts to copy a cursive *L* six times, diagonally

Age 11: Severe difficulties at all levels

Age 12: Severe difficulties with form, pattern, and reciprocity

Age 13: Student attempts to compensate by eliminating slanted lines

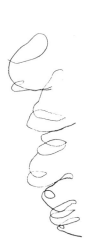

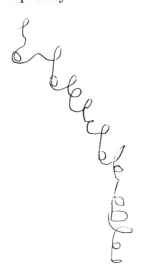

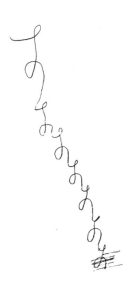

Age 12: Notice difficulty with directional shifts, especially on attempt #2. The third attempt was performed with extreme slowness.

Age 11: Student compensates by using extremely large forms.

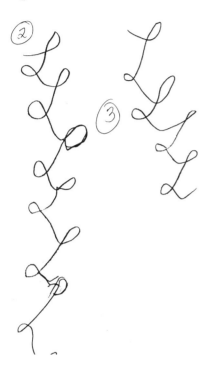

Five attempts to copy cursive *L* pattern

First attempt to copy *L* pattern by a 9-year-old non-dysgraphic student

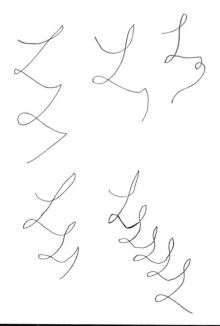

Pencil Grip Positions

A comfortable, efficient pencil grip is important; it increases fluency and decreases fatigue.

In an appropriate tripod pencil grip, the thumb and middle finger generally control the movement and the pointer finger controls pressure.

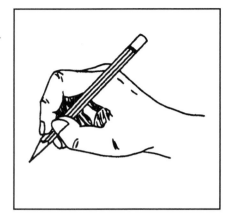

A left-handed tripod grip is the same as the right-handed grip; however, the paper slant is to the right.

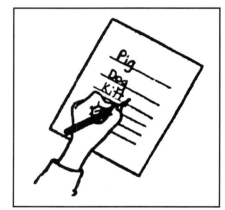

A left-handed grip can also use an inverted or "hook" position, with the paper slanted to the left.

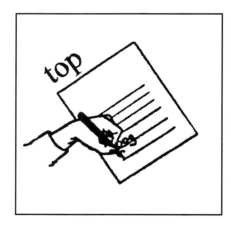

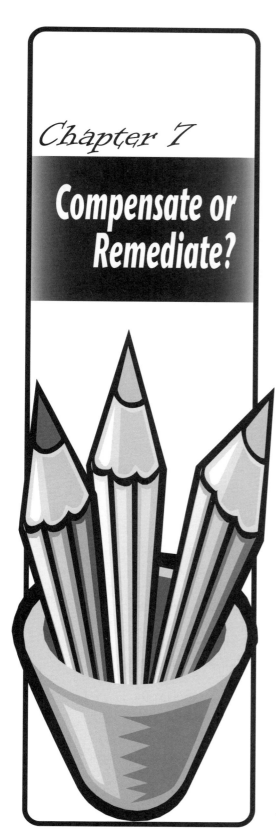

Chapter 7

Compensate or Remediate?

The overall goal in working with any student, particularly one who learns differently, is to help the student achieve success and enhance skills while maintaining positive feelings of himself as a learner. If a specific task is a struggle, the task may actually interfere with learning rather than help. For example, writing generally reinforces and consolidates information for a student. However, some students, especially those with dysgraphia, spend much more time on a written assignment than their classmates, but they learn less. Writing for them is a barrier to learning or demonstrating their knowledge. This requires interventions in the form of **compensations** or **remediation**. Compensations are techniques to bypass the problem and reduce the negative impact on learning. This is accomplished by avoiding the difficulty, changing the assignment or expectations, or using strategies to aid that particular aspect of the task. Compensations can also be called bypass strategies, or accommodations, the latter term used more frequently in legal situations. Remediation provides additional structured practice or reteaching of the skill or concept using specialized techniques to match the student's processing style and needs.

When a student struggles, the first and most essential step is to analyze the source of the student's confusion and/or difficulty. This is called the *breakdown point*. The breakdown point is that part of the task where the student begins to struggle or experience confusion. Once this point is determined, the teacher can then make a decision to provide either compensations or remediation. To determine the breakdown within a learning process, two questions are critical:

✔ Where is the breakdown occurring, i.e., what is the point where the student becomes confused or begins to struggle?

✔ What is the nature of the breakdown, i.e., what are the components of the task which are causing the confusion and/or struggle?

This essential information helps determine where to intervene as well as the appropriate method(s) needed to eliminate the confusion for the student. The goal is to change the task to enable the student to successfully learn the content or procedure being taught or to help the student fill in gaps within his development of the related skill.

Compensations

Compensations are utilized to alter how the information is presented to the student or how the student produces his response. For example, if a student has difficulty following continuous auditory input, a presentation rate modification can be used. The teacher would alter the presentation by speaking more slowly and stopping frequently to review and summarize the information. A production example of how to modify output for a student would be to warn her before calling on her in class, thereby providing more time for her to analyze the question and organize her answer. Another production example would be to allow a student more time on tests, again modifying the rate by allowing additional time. Mel Levine uses the term *bypass strategies*, and has identified nine ways to bypass problems encountered by students with learning differences. (Levine 1998, 592) These formats involve:

✔ Rate modification

✔ Volume reduction

✔ Complexity adjustment

✔ Prioritization

✔ Curriculum changes

✔ Special devices

✔ Alteration of routines

✔ Formal shifts

✔ Feedback modifications

Examples of how to modify the presentation form or production mode are presented in the summary on page 98. When modifications such as these examples are used, it is important to ensure that the student understands why a specific change or compensation is being used. The modification should not be embarrassing, nor should it imply lack of respect for the student. Some students may respond more comfortably if a trade is established. For example, the student may create a colorful computerized title page to be included with a shortened writing assignment.

Maintaining respect for the student and avoiding embarrassment, especially in front of peers, are vital. Use of a secret signal between the child and the teacher can be employed and all discussions should take place privately. The process of demystification should be continually used with students to reduce the mystery of what is going on while helping the student understand his own processing strengths and weaknesses. Demystification can also help the student understand his own goals and relate the task at hand to his own value system and goals for the future. It is important to assist the student in understanding his processing strengths as well as why and when specific modifications need to occur. This is a critical lifelong skill, and perhaps one of the most important, for any student who learns differently or struggles with some aspects of learning.

Many times students with dyslexia and/or dysgraphia are unsuccessful in the school environment because they do not know how or when to employ specific strategies to deal with a task. These students need to be taught how to learn in order to succeed not only in the school environment but also throughout life in managing a job or home activities. They need precise training in learning strategies and study skills. The three S's mnemonic can help keep in mind the necessary components. The three S's are **s**tructure, **s**ystematic, and **s**ensory to remind students to structure and organize the task, be systematic in their approach (proceed one step at a time), and use a variety of sensory systems or pathways.

Use of strategies is a critical step in teaching students to learn how to learn. Deshler defines a strategy as "a plan that not only specifies the sequence of needed actions but also consists of critical guidelines and rules related to making effective decisions during a problem-solving process." (Deshler 1996) A strategy, as a structured plan, often involves a plan to plan. Preplanning is one of the strategies most underused by dyslexic students, but it is also one of the most important compensations to help them deal with typical poor time management problems. With encouragement and continual reinforcement of the strategy, students can learn to use aids that will help them preplan. Their plan also needs to be very systematic (step by step) and involve multiple sensory pathways. Successful adult dyslexics find it critical to develop habits that rely on specific, structured strategies.

Remediation

Remediation involves intervention by the teacher and the most obvious is reteaching of the skill using more concrete or alternative methods. However, there are many other general types of remedial strategies that can be used at breakdown points. By understanding these types of interventions, a teacher can adapt almost any material and intervene for most problems demonstrated by a student. These interventions apply across nearly all curriculum areas and their use can greatly change the level of success a student experiences, her feelings of self-worth, and her belief in her own ability to learn. These nine general types of remedial assistance, as suggested by Levine (Levine 1998, 574) are listed on the summary on page 99:

✔ Automatization of subskills and/or neurodevelopmental function

✔ Scaffolding

✔ Design tasks that end at the breakdown point

✔ Separate breakdown points

✔ Staging

✔ Use multiple formats

✔ Deploy strengths and affinities

✔ Modeling

✔ Use of strategies

✔ Directed retraining

Throughout Part Two of this book, additional specific remedial strategies are discussed regarding skills for reading, spelling, writing, written expression, and memory tasks. Many times dyslexic students, while capable of learning skills and concepts, need to do so using alternate techniques. They respond best to multisensory methods and often need to be presented with the developmental steps explicitly rather than implicitly. The key is to incorporate the three S's: **s**tructure, **s**ystematic, and **s**ensory.

> **The 3 S's**
> - **S**tructure
> - **S**ystematic
> - **S**ensory

Deciding to Compensate or Remediate

When a student struggles, it is first necessary to identify the point in the task where his efficiency breaks down and confusion begins and thus identify the nature of the breakdown. The next step is to decide what to do at this breakdown point: compensate (modify or bypass) or remediate. This important decision, while seemingly simple, can be extremely complex because of its long-term implications.

The decision to **compensate** implies the belief that the student is unable to learn the skill or perform the task efficiently at that point in time, or ever. Therefore, it is necessary to create an alternate path to success. Spelling is a prime example because dyslexics generally do not develop automatic and efficient spelling. Use of a compensation such as a spell checker encourages the use of more complex words while increasing spelling accuracy in the final product. Some students, even those that learn to read efficiently, remain slow in their reading rate and fatigue easily. These students, especially in high school and college, benefit greatly from having their textbooks on tape. This frees them to focus on the primary task of comprehension and learning the concepts. Similarly, a computer is a vital compensation for many dyslexic and dysgraphic students because it enables them to concentrate more on the content of their writing.

Use of compensations should not mean that the basic task is totally avoided or ignored, especially for younger students. The student with poor spelling should be helped to develop as many skills as possible. The more phonetically logical their spelling is, the easier it will be to use a phonics-based spell checker, such as the Franklin Language Master®. Then, as eidetics (visual recognition skills) improve, they can progress to use of a spell checker on a computer. Students with poor and/or slow reading skills need to continue to practice reading, but should primarily do so with magazines and fun books, rather than difficult textbooks when the context is critical and the volume huge. Even the most severely dysgraphic student will need to write sometimes, and therefore, should have some writing practice. It is a significant detriment for these students to totally avoid all writing.

The primary goal of compensations is to provide a means whereby the student can continue to progress and develop conceptually without being held back because of the learning disability. Therefore, part of the decision to compensate can be based on the end goal of the task. For example, if the goal of a science test is to demonstrate knowledge of the content, it is unfair to count off for misspellings when the student has a true problem with spelling. If the goal is for the student to develop math understanding and competency, it is unfair to make him stay on multiplication practice because recall of the facts is not automatic. Rather, it is better to compensate for the unknown facts and allow the student to move on conceptually. At the same time, the student can continue to practice his times facts, but he should not be prevented from learning new concepts.

The decision to **remediate** implies the belief that the student is able to learn the skill and perform the task; however, a different, more systematic approach to the learning is needed. Part Two of this book is devoted to structured, multisensory, systematic techniques to remediate and enhance learning for students who learn differently.

Dealing with Frustrations

Students with learning difficulties experience frustrations throughout many, and sometimes all, of their academic tasks. They may struggle to understand, to produce information in a way that demonstrates when they do understand,

and to learn basic skills. Acknowledging the student's frustrations and how much harder she has to work is critical in helping the student realize that she is not dumb, weird, or strange for being so frustrated with the task. It is critical to reinforce the student's efforts and focus on areas of success. Helping the student deal with one subtask at a time is essential because it is often easier to be successful on one small part of a task even if the entire task appears overwhelming. One of the major teaching philosophies developed from the Gillingham remedial program, which was the first multisensory reading program developed specifically for dyslexics (Gillingham 1968), is to reinforce all successes and provide enough structure and intervention so that errors are kept to a minimum.

Even when substantial effort is spent helping a student structure the task to provide the greatest degree of success, there will still be times when the student becomes overwhelmed and is frustrated. It may occur within the process of learning to read, with study skill strategies, or with written assignments. It is critical for the student to know that this frustration is an integral part of the learning process, and it is normal for students to sometimes become overwhelmed. However, the student can also use strategies to decrease the feelings of being overwhelmed, the most important of which is breaking the task into smaller units. The student needs to realize that by focusing on just one small part at a time, he can achieve success with that small part and then go on to the next small part. Keep in mind, however, that students generally need help to learn how to break a task into subtasks.

Input to help students deal with frustration and feelings of being overwhelmed should be part of a demystification discussion to help the student understand his strengths and weaknesses. Pertinent examples and analogies relevant to the student's experiences and interest should be included. The following examples deal with concepts of struggling, experience, and mistakes, and can be adjusted or elaborated upon to fit the student's age and experience level.

Example one: The concept of struggling
"Struggling helps you build character, even though it may be more than you ever wanted, especially at this point in your life. This is because the brain learns by challenges. When you struggle, you are presenting your brain with some good challenges that help your brain grow, develop, and reorganize. Remember when you first learned to ride a bicycle . . . ?"

Depending on the student's age, inclusion of pictures of the brain and discussion of dendritic growth may be very useful. Some relevant brain books for children are Ellison 1995, Gupta 1997, and Simon 1997.

Example two: The concept of experience

"You can't expect to get this right the first time because you haven't practiced and you don't have experience. You can't be experienced until you go through the process often enough. Practice and experience help your brain pathways develop, grow, and get stronger."

If the student is nearing the age of interest in learning how to drive, a relevant example is the driver who automatically moves through the motions in comparison to the brand-new driver who must think about every step.

Example three: The concept of mistakes

"Mistakes help you learn. Without mistakes, you would never know which things need to be modified or changed. If you always did everything right, especially if you did it right the first time without any mistakes, how would you analyze the task or the process you are using?"

If the student is interested in athletics, examples of practicing moves for a particular sport or for dancing can be utilized.

Form of Bypass	Presentation Examples	Production Examples
Rate modification	• Stop frequently to review and summarize material • Speak slowly, with pauses after important information	• Warn student before requesting a verbal response (give a signal in advance) • Allow more time on tests
Volume reduction	• Highlight textbooks • Reduce reading load	• Allow shorter written reports
Complexity adjustment	• Give multiple practical examples of abstract concepts • Explain the abstract in concrete terms • Provide manipulative examples	• Give tests on one type of problem; don't mix problems • Student completes only one aspect of the task at a time • Create time line to complete longer projects and monitor consistently
Prioritization	• Emphasize key points to be learned from lesson • Provide an outline of lesson or procedure • Focus on one or two key aspects	• Grade only for content and not spelling • Have student focus on a single aspect of a writing assignment (i.e., elaboration)
Curriculum changes	• Reduce time in subjects requiring language processing • Provide breaks	• Let a child use print instead of cursive writing • Allow student to dictate answer to essay questions
Special devices	• Use reminder cards • Use wall chart of steps in assignment (staging) • Use books on tape	• Allow students to use a calculator, word processor, spell check, Franklin Language Master®, grammar check, outlining software
Alteration of routines	• Change subject schedules • Allow collaborative learning	• Permit breaks • Allow doodling • Encourage use of hands • Allow controlled movement during task
Formal shifts	• Show films • Allow experiential learning	• Use oral reports • Focus on recognition memory • Use portfolios • Allow credit for projects involving hands-on activities
Feedback modifications	• Provide encouragement while teaching	• Require self-rating • Private conferences • Modify grading

Modified from Levine 1998, 592

Interventions at Breakdown Points Summary

Intervention Type	Description/Examples
Automatization of subskills and/or neurodevelopmental function	• Practice at earlier learning stage; e.g., drill on math facts, sound/symbol associations • Enhance phonological awareness skills
Scaffolding	• Provide a structure within a task—report developer, mind map, or problem-solving plan • Use cloze procedures (fill-in-the-blank)
Design tasks that end at the breakdown point	• Accentuate a weak component by making it an end in itself; e.g., sorting out word problems by the process demanded • Use two colors of underlining; one for main idea and one for key facts • Use Post-its® to identify main idea in paragraph • Encourage paraphrasing
Separate breakdown points	• Slow down rate of speech • Verbalize at breakdown point; e.g., perform punctuation as a separate, verbalized step after writing the draft
Staging	• Organize tasks into manageable steps; e.g., separate writing into four steps: brainstorming, actual writing, application of mechanics, proofreading • Proofread in several distinct steps
Use multiple formats	• Present material in multiple ways/contexts; e.g., concept mapping, demonstration models, verbal summarization, synthesis
Deploy strengths and affinities	• Enable student to use strong pathways; e.g., learn math via demonstration models, improve comprehension by reading about special interests, verbalize nonverbal concepts, draw verbal concepts
Modeling	• Demonstration by teacher or other students • Have student demonstrate an operation at the breakdown point; e.g., show how to use a stepwise approach to a math problem
Strategy use	• Show student a technique to strengthen a breakdown point; e.g., rehearsal and self-testing techniques for studying
Directed retraining	• Reteach specific functions or skills; e.g., help a student develop a better pencil grip • Provide small group or individual review or tutoring

Modified from Levine 1998, 574

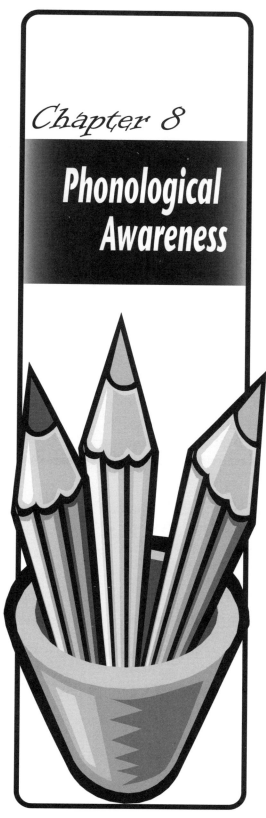

Chapter 8

Phonological Awareness

The discovery of the nature, importance, and necessity of phonological awareness and manipulations is the biggest breakthrough in reading pedagogy in this century. (Adams 1990; Reading Program Advisory 1996) An underlying awareness of speech sounds is critical to enable a student to discern patterns and sequences and to manipulate sounds within words. Students must be able to understand and have access to the sound structure of language. In 1994, Dr. Keith E. Stanovich, a leading reading expert from Canada, stated that our knowledge that "direct instruction in alphabetic coding facilitates early reading acquisition is one of the most well-established conclusions in all of behavioral science." (Stanovich 1994, 285-286) In 1995, Dr. G. Reid Lyon reported that 260 studies all converged on the finding that "the awareness of phonology is the core deficit for reading disabilities," a problem that affects 85% of our country's learning disabled children. (Lyon 1995)

Effective pre-reading instruction initiated early is the best way to increase literacy in our children. Because it is important to begin this development early, phonological awareness activities in preschool, kindergarten, and early elementary years are critical. Reading disabilities based on phonological awareness gaps can be remediated, although the percentage of success varies according to the researcher and method(s) used. Diamond and Mandel (1996) report that dyslexia identified in first or second grade may be remediated 82% of the time. Juel (1998) and Torgesen and Burgess (1998) report that less than one of eight (12½%) children who fail to read by the end of first grade will be at grade level by fifth grade. However, Diamond and Mandel (1996) also report that children identified in third to fifth grades may be remediated 46% of the time, and those identified later may only be treated successfully 10-15% of the time. While these statistics and reports are not consistent, the underlying message to teachers is clear: we need to start helping children solidify phonological awareness skills as early as possible. Additionally, phonological awareness gaps should receive focus in remedial programs for students of any age, as the importance of these skills cannot be ignored.

Definition

Our language system can be conceptualized as a hierarchical series of functions. At the highest level are components that help with meaning, grammatical structure and sentence connections. At the lowest level are phonological components. These enable us to distinguish the separate sounds that are embedded in words through our processing of distinctive sounds. This process of hearing and distinguishing sounds occurs independently from the process of dealing with letters and sound/symbol correspondence. Ideally, it also occurs prior to formal introduction of letters.

Phonological Awareness

Phonological awareness is the conscious awareness that words are composed of separate sounds.

- How many speech sounds in **grass**? (four sounds: /g/ /r/ /a/ /s/)
- How many speech sounds in **ox**? (three sounds: /o/ /k/ /s/)
- How many speech sounds in **yellow**? (four sounds: /y/ /e/ /l/ /o/)
- How many speech sounds in **once**? (four sounds: /w/ /u/ /n/ /s/)

This leads to the ability to identify and manipulate sounds within words.

- Say the sounds in these words in reverse order (note: this auditory activity deals only with sounds).

judge	(juj)	**kiss**	(sick)
votes	(stoev)	**peach**	(cheap)
time	(miet)	**meat**	(team)

- Say your name in "Pig Latin." (Move the initial sound [or blend] to the end of the word, and add the vowel sound /ay/.)

Regina (eginaray)	**Richards** (ichardsray)
John (onjay)	**Smith** (ithsmay or mithsay)

Phonological processing consists of a number of different processing tasks that encompass a wide range of skills. Phonological awareness is only one element of a whole level of language processing that is at the foundation of learning to use an alphabetic system. It is **not** phonics, but the ability to learn phonics is dependent on adequate phonological awareness.

The highest level of phonological awareness involves automaticity and an ability to self-correct errors in reading or spelling. It allows us to hold and compare our response to the printed word, judge our error(s), and make the correction. Without automatic phonological awareness, when we feel we have made an error (through meaning or other cues), we need to begin the laborious task of sounding out the word, step by step. With automatic phonological awareness, we can easily recognize and judge the mismatch caused by a letter omission, letter addition, sequence reversal, syllable omission, or other error, as in the examples on the next page.

- seep for *sleep*   (omission error)
- clop for *cop*   (addition error)
- clasp for *claps*   (reversal error)
- casual for *causal*   (reversal error)
- unstanding for *understanding*   (syllable omission error)

Information about all the letters in a word is obtained to match the word to the representation of the word stored in memory. This information is dependent upon accuracy of the phonological judgments. The stored images must represent all the letters for accurate word identification. Thus, efficient sight recognition is highly dependent on solid phonological awareness skills. Readers read the words by remembering how they read them previously. The term *sight* indicates that the sight of the word activates, in memory, information about the word's sounds, pronunciation, spelling, and meaning.

> . . . it has been proven beyond any shade of doubt that skillful readers process virtually each and every word and letter of text as they read. This is extremely counter-intuitive. For sure, skillful readers neither look nor feel as if that's what they do. But that's because they do it so quickly and effortlessly. Almost automatically, with almost no conscious attention whatsoever, skillful readers recognize words by drawing on deep and ready knowledge of spellings and their connections to speech and meaning.
>
> In fact, the automaticity with which skillful readers recognize words is the key to the whole system . . . . The reader's attention can be focused on the meaning and message of a text only to the extent that it's free from fussing with the words and letters. (Adams, 1998)

The Causal Connection

A strong causal connection exists between a child's awareness of sounds and learning to read. Phonological awareness is the understanding that spoken words and syllables are themselves made up of sequences of individual speech sounds. This understanding is essential for learning to read an alphabetic language where these elemental sounds or phonemes are represented by letters. Without phonological awareness, phonics will make no sense and the spelling of words can only be learned by rote. The best current theory of sight word learning proposes that readers learn sight words by forming connections between graphemes (letters) in the spellings and the phonemes underlying the pronunciation of individual words. (Torgesen 1999)

In the early stages of its development, phonological awareness does not involve written letters or words, and therefore, it is very different from what is traditionally called *phonics*. In later stages, work on phonological awareness and phonics can be mutually reinforcing. Therefore, phonological awareness abilities are critical prerequisites to reading and also a consequence of learning to read and practicing reading. At the lower end of the continuum, they are the critical prerequisites to reading. However, phonological awareness abilities at the higher end of the continuum, those that are more explicit, are primarily a result of the reading process. This is "the rich get richer" paradigm; students who have this skill develop even greater efficiency, and students who lack the skill become further and further behind their peers.

Early intervention is critical to help more students avoid this dilemma. The National Institute of Child Health and Human Development (NICHD) has been extremely active in supporting early intervention, based on over a decade of research.

> It is particularly distressing that government research shows that children can be identified as poor readers when they're as young as four or five, based merely on how they hear, remember, and repeat the subtle sounds found in everyday speech. Yet schools often don't jump on the problem until children are eight or nine.

> If a youngster does not receive special help until age nine, "it takes four times as long to move the same skill the same distance."

> "That means what could be addressed in 30 minutes a day in kindergarten now can take two hours a day by the fourth grade. The eighth grade teacher will have it even tougher with more ground to cover to even catch up—not to mention all the failure that the student has already experienced and the toll that takes on self-esteem." (Rubin 1997)

Research repeatedly shows that phonological awareness is a powerful predictor of success in learning to read. Some of the critical research findings include those here and on the following page:

- Phonological awareness is a most important core and causal factor separating normal and disabled readers. (Adams 1990; Share & Stanovich 1995)

- A preschooler's phonological aptitude predicts future skill at reading. (Yopp 1992; Lyon 1995)

- One of the best predictors of reading success in kindergarten and first grade is phoneme segmentation; young children who perform well on measures of phonological awareness are likely to be among the best readers. (Duane 1991)

- With current teaching and special education techniques, 74% of the children with reading disabilities at third grade will still be reading disabled in ninth grade. (Lyon 1996/97, 15)

- Phonological awareness abilities have a greater relationship to learning to read than do I.Q. factors, reading readiness, and listening comprehension. (Stanovich 1994; Lyon 1995)

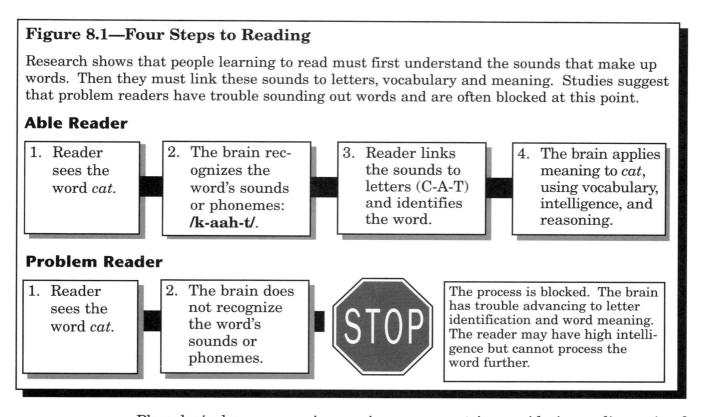

Figure 8.1—Four Steps to Reading

Research shows that people learning to read must first understand the sounds that make up words. Then they must link these sounds to letters, vocabulary and meaning. Studies suggest that problem readers have trouble sounding out words and are often blocked at this point.

Able Reader

| 1. Reader sees the word *cat*. | 2. The brain recognizes the word's sounds or phonemes: **/k-aah-t/**. | 3. Reader links the sounds to letters (C-A-T) and identifies the word. | 4. The brain applies meaning to *cat*, using vocabulary, intelligence, and reasoning. |

Problem Reader

| 1. Reader sees the word *cat*. | 2. The brain does not recognize the word's sounds or phonemes. | STOP | The process is blocked. The brain has trouble advancing to letter identification and word meaning. The reader may have high intelligence but cannot process the word further. |

Phonological awareness is a major component in considering a diagnosis of dyslexia. A phoneme, the smallest meaningful segment of spoken language, is a fundamental element of the linguistic system. Phonemes are important because they make up all spoken and written words. In our alphabetic language, different combinations of just 44 phonemes produce every word in the English language. Dyslexia represents a deficiency in processing these fundamental elements.

In the process of learning to read, the beginning reader must first come to a conscious awareness of the internal phonological structure of written words. Then he must realize that the sequence of letters on the page represents this phonological structure. (See Figure 8.1 on page 105, adapted from Holmes, 1997) With dyslexics, a deficit within the language system at this important phonological level often impairs the ability to automatically segment the written word into its underlying phonemic components. The word *cat* is one explosive sound, but it can be segmented into three underlying components: /k/ /a/ /t/. Without phonological awareness, exposure to print may be inefficient in fostering sound/symbol knowledge.

There are some children who may learn to read even with significant gaps at the level of phonological awareness, usually because they are visually skilled at remembering basic words and word configurations. However, their spelling is usually significantly impaired. In contrast, most students who begin school with little phonological awareness have trouble acquiring automatic alphabetic coding skill, and consequently, do not easily recognize words. When decoding is laborious, the end result is that reading for meaning is greatly hindered. When the process of word recognition demands too much cognitive capacity, there are fewer cognitive resources left to deal with the higher level process of comprehension. The opposite is the student who comes to school with an awareness of rhyme and alliteration. This student is at a higher level of readiness, which then has a powerful influence on his eventual success in learning to read and spell.

When students plod through learning to read with only minimal phonological manipulation skills, they struggle with comprehension, read slowly, and spell poorly. Their poor phonological manipulations can often be recognized by their struggles in tasks such as the following:

- Pig Latin (it is difficult or impossible)
- Segmenting a sound within a multi-syllabic word:
  Say industry without /d/   (*inustry*)
  Say encyclopedia without /p/   (*encycloedia*)
  Say encyclopedia without /l/   (*encycopedia*)
- Confusing similar words when speaking and/or writing:
  Pacific/specific
  reserve/reverse
  ephelant/elephant
  mazagine/magazine

Developmental Levels

Generalized areas of proficiency can be summarized into five types of activities. Students need facility in these tasks to enable the process of learning to read to be successful.

1. Retention of nursery rhymes
2. Compare and contrast sounds of words for rhyme and alliteration
3. Blending (/f/ /a/ /t/ is *fat*)
4. Segmenting (*fat* can be divided into three sounds and can be represented by three items such as fingers, blocks, or squares of felt.)
5. Phoneme manipulation (comparing, adding, deleting, and moving sounds)

Since this type of learning proceeds developmentally, there are expectations at particular levels. However, great variability exists among individual learners. Some may progress faster (or slower) than their peers.

The following listing delineates approximate student expectations at given levels:

Preschool Expectations

- Recall nursery rhymes and verses.
- Recognize rhyming.
- Complete a sentence using a predictable rhyming pattern, with cues provided by a picture and/or the sentence meaning.
- Distinguish separate sounds.
- Play with alliteration (*Silly Sally, boppy bunny*).
- Clap syllables (50% accuracy by age 4).
- Understand print concepts (know their way around books).

Kindergarten Expectations

- Produce a rhyming word for a given word.
- Recognize and produce alliteration.
- Clap syllables (90% accuracy by age 5).
- Count sounds in words. (How many sounds do you hear in *biz*?) (40-50% accuracy)
- Blend two sounds to make a word (/a/-/t/= *at*).
- Determine which of three words begins with the same sound as a target word (dog: mat, *dime*, top).*
- Determine which of three sounds begins with a sound that is different from the other two (ball, baby, *horse*).*
- Delete phonemes from words. (Say *pat*. Now say it again, but don't say /p/. [*at*])*
- Begin to substitute beginning sounds. (Change the /m/ in *mat* to /h/. [*hat*].)*

* by the end of the year

First Grade Expectations

- Demonstrate awareness of sounds and how print is organized.
- Understand that a word is comprised of sound units.
- Count sounds in words (*mat* = /m/-/a/-/t/). (70% accuracy by age 6)
- Recognize word family patterns and rhymes.
- Segment initial or final sounds in words. (What's the first sound you hear in *bat*?)
- Blend two to three phonemes (auditorily and visually).
- Can begin to make changes and represent these changes with a concrete object, such as a block. (If these two squares say /ot/, how would you make it say /pot/? *Add another block at beginning.*)
- Substitute beginning or ending sounds. (Change the *t* in *cat* to *p*. [*cap*])
- Hear and segment medial phonemes (by the end of the year).

Second Grade Expectations

- Demonstrate knowledge of most phonics elements (consonants, vowels, blends, clusters, syllables, common phonetic rules).
- Blend three to four phonemes (auditory and visually).
- Segment three to four phonemes, including words with blends.
- Spell phonetically.
- Delete a phoneme: take a sound out of a word and recombine sounds. (Say *meet*. Say it again, but don't say /m/. [*eet*])
- Perform more complex segmenting, blending, and transposition.
- Substitute syllables, representing changes in nonsense or real words, using a concrete object. (If these two squares say /rug-shun/, what chunk changes when we say /gum-shun/? *The first chunk changes.*)

Phonological Awareness Activity Suggestions in Developmental Order

The activity suggestions in Sections 8a, 8b, and 8c are in approximate developmental order. However, any given activity can be made easier or more complex by minor alterations. The overall purpose, especially at the beginning, is to help the student shift his attention away from the *content* of the language to its *form*. Awareness can be developed through a variety of games and activities that are brief, fun, and interspersed throughout the day. Games are an appropriate vehicle because they increase the student's level of involvement and enjoyment.

Caution:	These activities differ from traditional phonics games that use letter matching.

Since the goal of these tasks is to increase sensitivity to sounds within words, it is critical that students say the syllable patterns and words aloud as they progress through the activities. They do not derive the same benefit from silent speech; they need to kinesthetically feel the speech production while also hearing the sounds. If memory is an issue, some students may struggle to hold all the words in mind. In such situations, using picture cues can be helpful. Torgesen and Bryant's program, *Phonological Awareness Training for Reading,* begins all activities with picture cues. (Torgesen & Bryant 1994)

The following three sections present activity suggestions which can be used to teach or enhance skills at each level. The vocabulary used can be selected from any story or content topic that is currently relevant in the classroom. The suggestions may be modified or enhanced in a variety of ways and are intended as a suggestion or starting point to demonstrate the intended concept. Activities within any level may also be used to develop skills at the next or future levels, by modifying the task and increasing the challenge. This

---

Overview of the 9 Phonological Awareness Levels

Early Literacy Auditory Levels
- I.   Rhyming and Alliteration
- II. Sound Awareness and Rhyming Production
- III. Segmenting Sentences into Words

More Advanced Auditory Levels
- IV. Auditory Blending and Analysis
- V.   Syllable Segmentation
- VI. Phoneme Segmentation
- VII. Phoneme Manipulation

More Advanced Levels Integrating Auditory Activities with Letters/Words
- VIII. Syllable Manipulation
- IX. Higher Levels of Phoneme and Syllable Manipulation: Sound Games Using Vocabulary and Humor

---

flexibility is particularly useful in group activities where some students may benefit from more challenges than others. Similarly, an astute teacher may wish to simplify a task to help a given student achieve greater success and to practice a needed skill. While there is some progression in skill and difficulty within a level, the activities are not in rigid developmental order. At the higher, more advanced auditory levels, it is important to incorporate nonsense words. When students can automatically manipulate sounds in nonsense words, it is a sure sign that they can manipulate phonology.

These activities are not phonics, even though teachers often use phonics programs concurrently. However, when the goal is to develop phonological awareness, the activities designed to be purely auditory need to remain so and need to be performed without the use of letters. These activities cannot be embedded within other tasks, as the skills must be explicitly taught.

Chapter 8a: Phonological Awareness Early Literacy Auditory Levels

Activities in the three levels of the Early Literacy Auditory group are appropriate for preschool (levels 1 and 2), kindergarten, and first grade. However, many older students may have gaps at these levels and would also benefit from these activities.

Caution:	You can't fix phonological problems with a visual task.

Activity Suggestions

Level I. Rhyming and Alliteration

Activities in this auditory level focus on helping students appreciate sound patterns in language they hear. Students are helped to enhance their listening skills while identifying rhyme (words with identical ending sounds) and alliteration (words with identical beginning sounds). Activities in level one involve receptive skills for the students who primarily demonstrate their awareness through recognition. However, they may also say (verbally produce) a target word when given a picture or precise semantic cues.

1.1 Sound discrimination activities

- Place four different objects in four identical glass jars, varying the objects at different times. Example objects are wooden beads, a spoon, pebbles, and marbles. The children watch as the teacher demonstrates the sound of each by dropping the objects into a jar or shaking it. Then one child turns his back. Another student shakes a jar. The chosen student listens and tries to guess which sound he heard.

- Students each have a jar or other small container and five buttons. They close their eyes while the teacher slowly drops one to five buttons into a glass jar. Students open their eyes and, without looking at the teacher's jar, each selects the same number of buttons to drop in his own jar. As an alternative, students may indicate the number of buttons they heard by holding up that number of fingers.

1.2 Rhyme recognition activities

- Say two words and have student determine if they rhyme. (e.g., *go* / *top* [no], *my* / *buy* [yes])

- Say three words, two of which rhyme. Students determine which word is odd man out. (e.g., *mat, fat, nose* [*Nose* doesn't rhyme.])

1.3   Count words, repeating words modeled by teacher

- Have students repeat a sentence and then say it again while walking and saying one word with each step. *My name is Joe.* (four steps)

- Have students walk and repeat a set of rhyming words, saying one word per step. *ball, fall, tall* (three steps)

- As an alternative, students can jump once for each word in the sentence or rhyming set.

1.4   Incorporate games and activities using nursery rhymes and other stories or songs, discussing the words that rhyme

- Role-play, i.e., students can pretend to be Humpty Dumpty or Jack and Jill.

- Make models to match a story heard.

- Make puppets to match a story heard.

1.5   Recognize rhyming words when given a stimulus

- Example: after reading *What is that, said the cat?* (Maccarone 1995), ask, "What word sounds like *that* in the phrase *said the cat?*"

1.6   Read and discuss repetitive stories

- Example: *When it rains, it rains, and when it snows, it snows.* (Martin 1970)

1.7   Fill in the word that rhymes, using context and picture clues

- Example from a story with picture and context cues: "Open it up," said the pup. "How?" said the cow. "I'll use force," said the _____. (*horse*). (Maccarone 1995)

1.8   Create silly words using rhyme and alliteration as names for puppets, animals, dolls, or creative drawings

- Examples: Silly Billy, Dino the Rhino, Happy the hopping Hippo

1.9 **Sing nursery rhymes and songs and substitute words to play with the words and make additional rhymes. Substitutions should be provided by the adult.**

Example: "Twinkle, Twinkle Little Star" can be changed to "Twinkle, Twinkle Little Car."

Level II. **Sound Awareness and Rhyming Production**

Activities in this auditory level focus on continuing to enhance the students' awareness of sounds and help them manipulate sounds for rhyming. At the beginning, sufficient picture and semantic cues may be provided to help students rhyme, but these cues are faded out as students become more proficient. At this level, they also begin to use manipulatives (not letters) to represent sounds or sound patterns.

Caution:	Always use a letter sound, not a letter name. Be careful to pronounce each consonant clearly, without adding /uh/ to the sound.

2.1 **Fill in the word that rhymes, using books that place the rhyming word or picture cue on a following page. Encourage students to predict what the word will be before turning the page.**

- Example from: *Is Your Mama a Llama?* (Guarino 1989)
  "She's got flippers and whiskers and eats fish all day . . .
  I do not think llamas act quite in that way.
  Oh, I said, I'm beginning to feel
  that your mama must really be a . . . . (*seal*)"

2.2 **Have students complete poems/rhymes by inserting a word that rhymes, based on the meaning of the sentence. Provide cues as needed.**

Example:
There is an eyeball in the gumball machine
Right there between the red and the green
Lookin' at me as if to say
You don't need any more gum _____ (*today*) (Silverstein 1981, 68)
(cue if needed: /t/ or /too/)

2.3 Read poems that use made-up rhyming words (*Animaloo*) and then help students create their own nonsense word.

Example:

I got grabbed by the elk and the caribou
They tied me up with a vine lasso
And whisked me away to *Animaloo*,
Where they locked me up in the People Zoo
(Silverstein 1996, 80)

2.4 Create rhymes using manipulatives. Students may use blocks or chips at their desks while you use large felts in the front of the room, or they may stand and hold large pieces of construction paper. This is an auditory activity that uses a color to represent a word part. In the examples below, the letter in the circle represents a color. The color itself is not associated with any given sound, but rather is used to represent *sameness* or *difference*.

- We're going to use these two circles to represent sounds we hear. Let's use Mary's name. The first sound is /m/ and we'll use the red circle. What are the rest of the sounds in *Mary*? Right, /ary/. We'll show these with a yellow circle:

  Ⓡ   Ⓨ
  M   ary   (*Mary*)

Let's change /m/ (point to Ⓡ in Mary) to /b/ (select a new color, Ⓖ).

What do we have now?

  Ⓖ   Ⓨ
  B   ary   (*Bary*)

Right, now we have *Bary*—that rhymes with *Mary*.

What else could we use to rhyme with *Mary* and *Bary*?

Student: Change /b/ (point to Ⓖ) to /sh/ (points to Ⓦ):

  Ⓦ   Ⓨ
  Sh   ary   (*Shary*)

Good, now we have *Shary, Bary*, and *Mary*. They all rhyme.

2.5 Use rhyming words to complete a sentence.
  - Use words all from the same category. For example, have students think of all color words:
    So crisp and clean
    These leaves are ____. (*green*)
    See the funny clown
    He's all dressed in ____. (*brown*)

  - Omit the category cue and have students complete the sentence:
    Isn't he funny,
    He hops like a ____. (*bunny*)
    From high on the steeple,
    We saw many ____. (*people*)

2.6 Teach location words *start* and *end*, using a train analogy. Give the children a picture or model of a train with an engine, freight car, and caboose.
  - Begin using the terms *start* and *end*, and point out the appropriate locations on the train. Have the children take turns being the *start* sound (engine) or *end* sound (caboose). Use their names, asking, "Who else has a name that starts with the /j/ sound?" (Jane stands up and becomes the engine). "Right, *Jane* has the start sound /j/. Okay, now the end sound in Jane is /n/. Who else has a name that ends in /n/? Good. *Ken*, you can be the caboose." (If desired, two or three other students can be in the middle and the *train* can chug around for a minute or two before the students return to their seats.)

  - If desired, teach that the *start* sound is the same as the *first* sound.

  - The teacher says a word such as *cat* and asks if the /k/ sound is at the *start* or *end* position of the word. Students may respond by pointing to the corresponding car on the train.

  - The teacher also asks students, "Think about sounds that words end with. Does *mermaid* end with /d/ or /s/?" (Provide choices.)

2.7 Teach the term *middle* using a variety of manipulatives and the above train game.

2.8 Sound matching activities. Teacher asks questions such as the following:

- Do *pin* and *pipe* start with the same sound?
- Do *dog* and *pig* end with the same sound?
- Do *cat* and *mouse* end with the same sound?

2.9 Purely auditory sound isolation activities. Teacher asks questions such as the following:

- What's the first sound (or *start* sound) in *rose*?
- What's the last sound in *cat*?
- Tell me which of these words end with the /t/ sound: *sad* (no), *heat* (yes), *bat* (yes), *fish* (no), *kit* (yes)
- Do these words have the /g/ sound in the middle? *August* (yes), *swing* (no), *sugar* (yes), *hamburger* (yes), *forgive* (yes), *goodness* (no)

2.10 Sound isolation activities using manipulatives

- Give each student a piece of colored construction paper. Three students who are holding different colors come to the front. Tell the class that these colors represent the sounds in the word *fun*. Give the following directions:
  ✔ Point to the student who has the first sound in *fun*. (Students point.)
  ✔ Say the first sound. (/f/)
  ✔ Point to the end sound in *fun*. (Students point.)
  ✔ Say the end sound. (/n/)
  ✔ Point to the middle sound in *fun*. (Students point.)
  ✔ Say the middle sound. (/u/)
  ✔ Now, let's say all the sounds in order: /f/-/u/-/n/ *fun*. (Students repeat as teacher taps students in order.)

  The goal of these activities is awareness; the teacher segments and students repeat.

2.11 Phoneme counting activities: recognition level

At this recognition level, it is acceptable if students cannot yet completely separate each sound. Assist as necessary.

- There are three sounds in the word *meet*. Let's walk (or march), taking one step for each sound in *meet*.
- (Choose three students to come to the front.) These students represent the sounds in *dog* (or any consonant-vowel-consonant word). "Let's see if we can figure out the

The Source for Dyslexia & Dysgraphia
Copyright © 1999 LinguiSystems, Inc.

sounds. What's this sound? /d/ What's this sound? /o/ and what's this sound? /g/." (Tap one student per sound.) Students stand about a foot apart and repeat the sounds: /d/-/o/-/g/.

- *Push* the students together and say, "Now we have /d/-/o/-/g/ together. That says *dog*."

2.12 Word sort activities using pictures (not letters)
- Using pictures, sort by initial consonant sound.

  Make two columns, one with a picture of a *dog* and one with a picture of a *cat*.

  Give students pictures of common objects that start with either of the target sounds, /d/ or /k/.

  Have students place a picture in the appropriate column, saying the word and the target word, such as *"Donut* starts like *dog."*

- Vary the activity using different beginning target sounds.

- Vary the activity using three columns.

- Vary the activity, having students sort by ending consonant sound.

- The activity is easier with consonant-vowel-consonant words (**m**at, to**p**). The activity is harder with words that begin or end in blends (**st**op, pu**mp**).

2.13 Odd man out: auditory tasks
- What word starts with a sound that is different from the start of the other words? *bag, nine, beach, bike* (*nine*)

  (If this is too difficult, only give students three choices.)

- What ends with a different sound? *hot, pop, hop, mop* (*hot*)

- What has a middle sound that is different? *mat, pat, sat, mitt* (*mitt*)

- Say a silly sentence, such as *Sally smiles sweetly at Sue*. Ask, "Which word does not start with the /s/ sound?" (*at*)

Level III. Segmenting Sentences Into Words
Activities at this auditory level focus on helping students perceive word boundaries. This important auditory analytic task is critical for later development of syllabification skills. Students use manipulatives and kinesthetic activities to represent and reinforce their awareness of separate words.

> **Caution:** These activities differ from traditional phonics games that use letter matching.

3.1 Count words using concrete manipulatives and kinesthetic activities.

- Student uses blocks to represent each word in the sentence, "My dog is Fluffy." (Figure 8a.1)

Figure 8a.1

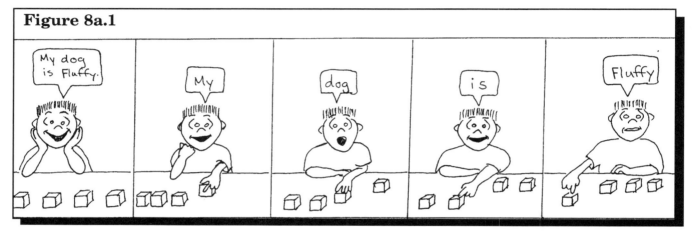

- Say a sentence such as *I like cookies and milk.* Have the students walk (or march), taking one step for each word in the sentence. They should say each word as they take the corresponding step.

- (Choose four students to come to the front.) "These students represent the words in the sentence, *My cat is orange.* Let's see if they can figure out their words." The first student takes one step forward and says *my*. The second student takes one step forward and says *cat*. Continue.

3.2 Orally segment sentences into words.
- Sitting in a circle, each child says one word in a familiar nursery rhyme such as "Mary Had a Little Lamb."

- Sitting in a circle, one student throws a ball to another. The student holding the ball says the next word in a familiar rhyme, poem, or song.

- The teacher (or student) says a sentence and students clap, repeat, or tap the table, matching one clap to each word.

3.3 **Use counting, clapping, or tapping to identify individual words in familiar written sentences, songs, or stories. Students are NOT requested or required to read the words, only identify them as individual words.**

- The teacher puts a poem or story on a story board, and the children take turns pointing to each word and counting. (Figure 8a.2)

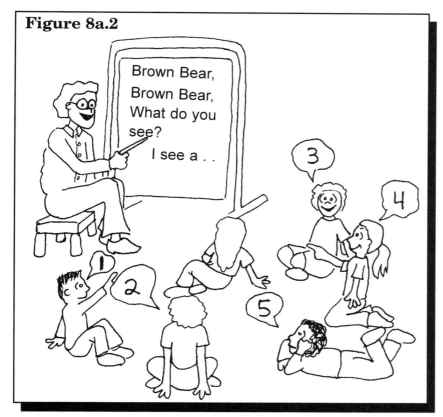

Figure 8a.2

Brown Bear,
Brown Bear,
What do you
see?

I see a . .

3.4 **Identify missing words from a list.**

- Listen to these words: *goosebumps, adventure, peaceful.* Now I'll say them again but I'll leave out one. You tell me which one I left out: *adventure, peaceful.* (*goosebumps*)

- As a variation, use a sentence rather than isolated words.

- Listen: *The peddler saw the monkey.*

  Listen again and tell me what's missing: *The peddler saw the _____* or *The _____ saw the monkey.*

3.5 **Use body movements to indicate or demonstrate words in sentences.**

- Students determine the number of words in a sentence the teacher or another student says. That number of students come to the front. For example, given *The goat runs*, three students come forward.

- One student stands and says *the*.

- The next student says *goat* and pretends to be a goat.

- The third student role-plays *runs*.

3.6 Use simple signs or sign language to represent each word in a sentence.

3.7 Combine alliteration with word counting.
- The teacher says an alliterated phrase and students count the words using clapping or tapping. After counting, the teacher asks, "Do you hear the same sound at the beginning of each word? What is it?"

    fat furry friend (3)

    silly sister Sally (3)

- The children make up silly phrases that use alliteration and then count the words. Incorporate the use of concrete manipulatives and role playing as relevant.

    kitty cat comes clean (4)

    pretty Polly parrot (3)

Chapter 8b: Phonological Awareness More Advanced Auditory Levels

Level IV. **Auditory Blending and Analysis**

The auditory blending activities help students identify the beginnings and endings of words, and eventually the middle parts. They also learn to pull sounds together as they progress to more advanced levels of phonological awareness. It is important that all of these activities be performed in an auditory mode, although manipulatives and kinesthetic movements may be used to help make tasks more concrete and/or more fun.

Initially, these activities should primarily involve recognition tasks, where the students are given a choice of two or three words from which to select the answer. Later on, ideally in kindergarten, the students can begin to retrieve, or generate, the answer on their own.

Caution:	Always use the letter sound, not the letter name. Sounds are indicated by / /.

4.1 **Word games with syllable and phoneme blending**
- What do I have if I put these together?
  ham   *bur*   *ger*
  un   *der*   *cov*   *er*
- What do I have if I put these together?
  /s/   /a/   /t/
  /gr/   /ā/   /t/

4.2 **Sound isolation activities**
- All children whose names start with /m/ may go line up.
- Let's see if we have any children whose names start with the same sound as Billy's name.
- Ask students if they hear a given sequence of sounds within another word:
      Do you hear *bat* in *rabbit*?
      Do you hear *part* in *apartment*?

4.3 **Song "If You Think You Know This Word" (Yopp 1992, 699)**

Tune: "If You're Happy and You Know It, Clap Your Hands" 🎵

If you think you know this word, shout it out!

If you think you know this word, shout it out!
If you think you know this word,
You can tell me what you've heard,
If you think you know this word, shout it out!
(Teacher says a segmented word such as /k/-/a/-/t/,
and children respond by saying the blended word /kat/.)

4.4 Position of consonant blends or digraphs activity

- The teacher says three words containing a given blend or digraph. The teacher then repeats each word and has the children determine the position of the target blend. The train analogy may be used to reinforce the meaning of beginning, middle, end in each word.

- Example dialogue: "Listen carefully to these words. They all have the sounds /st/ in them. Listen for /st/ in *fist, stamp, understand*. Is the /st/ in *fist* at the beginning, in the middle, or at the end?

- Example sets of words.
  st — fi**st**, **st**amp, under**st**and
  th — fa**th**er, bo**th**, **th**ose
  sh — fi**sh**ing, **sh**oes, pu**sh**
  tr — **tr**icks, coun**tr**y, **tr**ain

- As a variation, children can use manipulatives to indicate the position of the target sound(s). For example, place three pieces of colored paper in a line on the board: green, white, and red. Give each student the same three colors. Explain that students are to hold up the green paper if the sound is at the beginning, the white paper if it's in the middle, and the red paper if the sound is at the end of the word. One student may then come to the board and point to the position of the target blend in the word teacher says.

Caution:	It is much easier for students to identify the beginning and ending sounds. The medial sounds are more challenging.

Definition: A consonant blend is defined as two or three consonants that work together within a syllable, with each retaining its own sound. For example, fi**rst**, **spl**ash, and re**se**n**tm**ent. It is important for students to recognize that the sounds within a blend can be separated, as this is critical for accurate spelling.

Definition: Diagraphs (or digraphs) are two letters that make only one sound. For example, mu**sh**, **ph**one, **ch**ip, **th**at.

4.5 Sing songs that play with phonemes or that substitute words and word parts in a rhyming pattern. Remember to say the phoneme or sound and not the letter name. (Yopp 1992, 700)

Example song: "Who has a /d/ word to share with us?" 🎵

Tune: "Jimmy Cracked Corn and I Don't Care"

Who has a /d/ word to share with us?
Who has a /d/ word to share with us?
Who has a /d/ word to share with us?
It starts with the /d/ sound!

[One student says *dog*.]

Dog is a word that starts with /d/.
Dog is a word that starts with /d/.
Dog is a word that starts with /d/.
Dog starts with the /d/ sound.

Example song: "What's the sound that starts these words?" (This can be varied to use medial and final sounds.) 🎵

Tune: "Old MacDonald Had a Farm"

Initial:
What's the sound that starts these words:
Turtle, time, and *teeth*?
(Wait for a response from the children.)
/t/ is the sound that starts these words:
Turtle, time, and *teeth.*
With a /t/, /t/ here, and a /t/, /t/ there,
Here a /t/, there a /t/, everywhere a /t/, /t/.
/t/ is the sound that starts these words:
Turtle, time, and *teeth.*

What's the sound that starts these words:
Chicken, chin, and *cheek*?
(Wait for a response from the children.)
/ch/ is the sound that starts these words:
Chicken, chin, and *cheek.*

With a /ch/, /ch/ here, and a /ch/, /ch/ there,
Here a /ch/, there a /ch/, everywhere a /ch/, /ch/.
/ch/ is the sound that starts these words:
Chicken, chin, and *cheek.*

What's the sound that starts these words:
Daddy, duck, and *deep?*
(Wait for a response from the children.)
/d/ is the sound that starts these words:
Daddy, duck, and *deep.*
With a /d/, /d/ here, and a /d/, /d/ there,
Here a /d/, there a /d/, everywhere a /d/, /d/.
/d/ is the sound that starts these words:
Daddy, duck, and *deep.*

You all did great, so clap your hands!
(clap, clap, clap, clap, clap)

Medial:
What's the middle sound in these:
Leaf and *deep* and *meat?*
(Wait for a response from the children.)
/ee/ is the middle sound in these:
Leaf and *deep* and *meat.*
With a /ee/, /ee/ here, and a /ee/, /ee/ there,
Here a /ee/, there a /ee/, everywhere a /ee/, /ee/.
/ee/ is the middle sound in these:
Leaf and *deep* and *meat.*

Final:
What's the sound that ends these words:
Duck and *cake* and *beak?*
(Wait for a response from the children.)
/k/ is the sound that ends these words:
Duck and *cake* and *beak.*
With a /k/, /k/ here, and a /k/, /k/ there,
Here a /k/, there a /k/, everywhere a /k/, /k/.
/k/ is the sound that ends these words:
Duck and *cake* and *beak.*

4.6 **Create your own sound awareness activities using
nursery rhymes or familiar stories.**
Note: It is easier to first identify position of continuant

sounds such as /z/, /s/, /sh/, /f/, /s/. Noncontinuant sounds are more difficult, such as /d/, /t/, /g/, /k/, /ch/.

Level V. **Syllable Segmentation**

These auditory activities help the students advance into more elaborate activities focusing on syllables. Students learn to listen for the *chunks* within words and begin to understand that each syllable must contain a *talking vowel* (a vowel that carries a sound). Pictures and manipulatives may be used for any of these activities to help make the task more concrete and lessen the memory load. When progressing through each activity, begin with the simplest tasks and progress to greater challenges. The progression to use (in order of difficulty) is:
- compound words
- two-syllable words
- words of three and more syllables

5.1 **Syllable recognition: teacher models a word said in syllables. Students repeat the word in syllables and then blend the syllables into a word.**
- The teacher says a multi-syllabic word with a one-second pause between the syllables, e.g., *tea-cher.*
- Students repeat: *tea-cher.*
- Students say the word without a pause: *teacher.*

5.2 **Humming: students repeat a word said by the teacher and then hum the word to identify the number of chunks within that word.**
Examples:
goosebumps (2)   *detective* (3)
adventure (3)   *undercover* (4)

5.3 **Syllable identification and naming: students segment individual words into syllables, matching a movement to each syllable while saying the syllable.**
- Clap once for each syllable, saying the syllable while making each clap. (Refer to Figure 8b.1 on page 126.)
- Tap the table once for each syllable, saying the syllable during each tap.
- Jump once for each syllable, saying the syllable during each jump.
- Put your hand flat under your chin and say the word in syllables. Feel the downward movement of your chin as

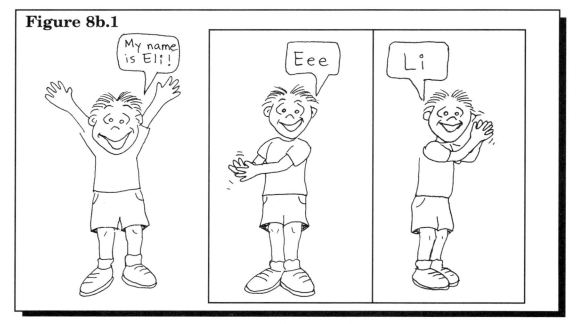

Figure 8b.1

each syllable is said, counting the syllables with the fingers on your other hand.

- Using Unifex Cubes® (or other manipulatives that hook together), display three cubes and say, "This represents the three parts, or the syllables, in the word *jellyfish*. Who can separate these cubes while telling us each syllable?"

  Vary the activity using one-, two-, three-, and four-syllable words.

  Vary the activity by saying a word and having a student select the correct number of cubes.

5.4 Sorting activities: sort pictures of words by the number of syllables

- Make three columns on the chalkboard, numbering each 1, 2, or 3.

- Place facedown a set of simple picture cards representing words of one to three syllables.

- Student selects a picture, claps or taps the number of syllables in the word, and places the picture under the corresponding number (using masking tape on a chalkboard or a magnet on a magnetic board).

- Variation: add columns 4 and 5 and pictures of four- and five-syllable words as students progress.

Sequence: progression of difficulty for syllable deletion tasks (for Activities 5.5 and 5.6)

✔ Delete initial or final syllable in compound words, using cubes.

✔ Delete initial or final syllable in two-syllable words, using cubes.

✔ Delete initial or final syllable in three-syllable words, using cubes.

✔ Delete initial or final syllable auditorily, without using cubes.

✔ Delete medial syllable, using cubes.

✔ Delete medial syllable auditorily.

5.5 Syllable deletion activities with blocks

• This activity uses different cubes or blocks to represent each syllable. Have students actually remove the cube as they omit the syllable. Examples:

Say *snowman*. (Student says the word and places out two blocks.) Say it again, but don't say *snow*. (Student removes the first block and says *man*.)

Tell me what *chalkboard* is without *board*.

Tell me *cucumber* without saying *cu*.

5.6 Syllable deletion activities

• Say a word and have students repeat it. Ask students to say it again, omitting one syllable. Begin with compound words and progress to two-syllable words.
  Examples:
  Say *cowboy*. Say it again, but don't say *boy*. *(cow)*
  Say *spaceman*. Say it again, but don't say *space*. *(man)*
  Say *goosebumps*. Say it again, but don't say *bumps*. *(goose)*
  Say *bubble*. Say it again, but don't say *ble*. *(bub)*

• As students progress, longer words may be used.
  Say *capturing*. Say it again, but don't say *cap*. *(turing)*
  Say *polkadot*. Say it again, but don't say *dot*. *(polka)*
  Say *undercover*. Say it again, but don't say *der*. *(uncover)*
  Say *helplessly*. Say it again, but don't say *less*. *(helply)*

5.7 Play a card game: Syllable War

• Use a deck of simple picture cards representing words with one to five syllables.

• Deal the cards evenly to two students who place them picture side down in a pile.

• Each player turns over his top card and counts the syllables in the word.

• The player with the largest number of syllables takes the exposed cards.

- A *syllable war* occurs if both players have words containing the same number of syllables. At that point, each player calls, "Syllable war!" and places one card from his pile facedown in the center. He then turns over the next card, and the student with the largest number of syllables pictured in the turned over card wins all the cards.

- As a variation, three or four students can play, using a larger stack of picture cards.

5.8 Syllables within words

Teacher: Is the word *rain* in *rainbow*?

Student: (claps *rainbow*, saying each syllable as he claps it.) Yes

Teacher: Is the word *danger* in *gingerbread*?

Student: (claps *gingerbread*, saying each syllable as he claps it.) No

Level VI. Phoneme Segmentation

These auditory activities help the students break words into their individual sounds and make more advanced auditory judgements about sounds within words. These more elaborate activities focus on individual sounds without using letter cues. Pictures and manipulatives may be used for any of these activities to simplify the task and decrease the memory load.

Caution:	It is difficult to teach auditory judgements using visual letters.

6.1 Strategies for students having difficulties segmenting sounds

- Start with chopping the word into two parts. Example: "I'm going to show you a way of saying words in parts— then you try it." The larger chunks carry more meaning and may be easier for some students. Note: be sure to say the letter sound, not its name.

  pat: /p/+/at/
  kit: /k/+/it/
  coat: /coa/+/t/
  sleep: /sl/+/ee/+/p/

- When students are successful, progress into chopping a word into its individual sounds.
     pat: /p/+/a/+/t/
     let: /l/+/e/+/t/
     meet: /m/+/ee/+/t/
     sleep: /s/+/l/+/ee/+/p/

- Provide extra practice in having students isolate the initial or final sound, if necessary.

- Use iteration of the sound; some students need to hear a sound emphasized in order to separate the initial sound. Explain that the word is like a rubber band. We can stretch it out like this: ssss-at.

     This does not work with stop consonants (b, p, t, d, k, g), as in b, b, b, b, b, bat or t, t, t, t, t, telephone.

     Have students stretch out the first sound in their names, if appropriate.

     Isolate and stretch out appropriate final sounds.

- Perform sound isolation tasks first as a recognition task and later as a retrieval task.
     Recognition: What sound do you hear first in *dog*? /d/ or /m/? (/d/)

     Retrieval: What sound do you hear first in *dog*? (/d/)

6.2 Segment words into sounds.
- Students actively segment words into component sounds using manipulatives, matching each movement to the vocalization of each sound.

- Using one-syllable words, have the student say each word slowly, separating the phonemes and marking each sound. *Cat* has three taps: /k/ /a/ /t/.
     Example:
     Fist patterns (using fist to tap the table).

     Use rhythm sticks or other percussion instrument to beat out each sound.

     Tap blocks or colored squares for each sound.

     Lift a finger for each sound.

6.3 Sound to word matching
- Is there a /k/ in *bike*?

- Is there /m/ in *bike*?

6.4 Sound deletion activities: deletion of isolated sounds

- Say *cat*. What is left if /k/ is removed from *cat*? (*at*)

- Say *seat*. Say *seat* again without /t/. (*sea*)

- What sound do you hear in *meet* that is missing from *eat*? (/m/)

- What sound do you hear in *door* that is missing from *or*? (/d/)

6.5 Deletion of sounds within blends

Use only after students have thoroughly mastered Activity 6.4. Blends with /r/ and /l/ are most difficult.

- Say *stick*. Now say it again, but don't say the /t/ sound. (*sick*)

- Say *pump*. Now say it again, but don't say /m/. (*pup*)

- Say *stake* without /s/. (*take*)

- Say *stake* without /t/. (*sake*)

- Say *past* without /t/. (*pas*)

- Say *past* without /s/. (*pat*)

If students struggle to separate the sounds within a blend, encourage them to say the blend slowly, focusing on what they *feel* their mouths doing as they start the blend, and then again as they finish the blend. Omission of the sound on the *outside* of the blend is easiest, as /s/ in *stop* or /p/ in *clasp*.

6.6 Comparison of sounds within words, using manipulatives

- Students use blocks. The teacher may use felt squares on a felt board. Have one student at a time work at the board, while the others work at their desks. When using colors, a specific color only represents sameness within the pattern.

    R **W** **G** This represents *mip*. Which sound changes when we say *kip*? (*the first*)

    B **W** **G** Because we changed the first sound, we change the first block. Any color is okay. The colors do not have a sound, unless we're using the same sound in our word. Now *touch* and *say kip*. (Student touches each block while saying its sound—/k/+/i/+/p/.) Good. Now let's change *kip* to *kik*. (Student touches and says *kip*.) Let's see, *kip*, *kik*. The end changes.

(Student takes out **G** and puts in **B**: **B** **W** **B**)

Teacher: Now touch and say again. (Student does so.) Why do you have two of the same color?

Student: Because I hear /k/ at the beginning and at the end.

See Figure 8b.2 for an example comparing *hat* and *rat*.

- Build a long chain, using dialogue as above. Make only one change each time: substitute, add, or omit a sound. Model changes as needed. The primary goal is for students to recognize the sounds and segment individual sounds from the pattern. Example chain:

shook **R** **B** **W**

took **G** **B** **W**

tak **G** **Y** **W**

tam **G** **Y** **R**

tamp **G** **Y** **R** **W**

Figure 8b.2

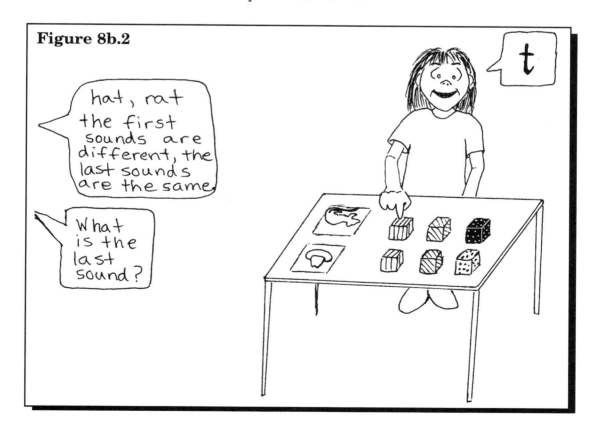

samp **B** **Y** **R** **W**

sap **B** **Y** **W**

- Students use construction paper.
  Say a word such as *run*. Students determine the word has three different sounds. Three students holding different colors come to the front. The teacher says, "How do we change *run* to *fun*?" Students decide the first student leaves (representing /r/) and a new color comes in (to represent /f/).

6.7 **Sing a song, "Listen, Listen to my Word" to the tune of "Twinkle, Twinkle, Little Star." (Yopp 1992, 702)** ♫

Tune: "Twinkle, Twinkle, Little Star"

(*chorus*) Listen, listen to my word,
Then tell me all the sounds you heard: *race*.
(Students say /r/+/a/+/s/.)

(*slowly*) /r/ is one sound,
/a/ is two,
/s/ is last in *race*, it's true.

(*chorus*) Listen, listen to my word,
You told me all the sounds you heard.

(*chorus*) Listen, listen to my word,
Then tell me all the sounds you heard: *coat*.
(Students say /k/+/o/+/t/.)

(*slowly*) /k/ is one sound,
/o/ is two,
/t/ is last in *coat*, it's true.

(*chorus*) Listen, listen to my word,
You told me all the sounds you heard.

(*chorus*) Listen, listen to my word,
Then tell me all the sounds you heard: *go*.
(Students say /g/+/o/.)

(*slowly*) /g/ is one sound,
/o/ is two,

And that is all in *go,*
It's true.

Thanks for listening
To my words
And telling all the sounds you heard!

6.8   Secret pictures game: large group activity
- This game requires that students both segment and blend sounds.

- Give a child a picture of an object, the name of which is a common three-letter word. The child keeps the picture (and name) a secret.

- The child segments the word aloud for the group (e.g., /k/+ /i/+/ng/).

- The group blends the sounds together and tries to guess the word. (*king*)

- To increase the challenge, the students can be given a code to use, such as the MFR key words. (See Chapter 9.)
  e.g., The word I'm thinking of contains the beginning sounds of these words: *doll, on, goat.*
  (/d/+/o/+/g/: *dog*)

6.9   Round   robin—change   that   sound: large   group activity
- Students sit in a circle. The teacher says a word and demonstrates how to change the word by substituting the ending sound (*hit* ➔ *him)*. The first student uses the last word he heard and changes the ending consonant (*him* ➔ *hip)*.

- After changing several words based on one stimulus, switch the stimulus word, or have students change the middle or the beginning sound.

- Provide models as needed for each different type of change.

- As students learn the procedures, have the students hold a *change that sound* ball as they take a turn. The student passes the ball to any student, who then has the turn.

6.10 Use a "sound of the day."
- The teacher selects a given sound, such as /m/. Throughout the day, all children's names will be changed

so that the first sound is substituted with the /m/ sound. For example, *Regina* becomes "mĭ-gina," *Sue* becomes "moo," and *George* becomes "morj."

6.11 Use riddles.

- The students listen to a riddle, give the answer word, act out the word, and then spell the word orally, sound by sound. As students develop skill, they can compose their own riddles. It is easier if the sounds are presented in their correct sequence, and much more challenging if the sequence is changed.

- "I am thinking of a name of an animal. Its middle sound is /o/. It begins with a /d/, it ends with a /g/. What's the word?" (*dog*)

6.12 If students are also (but separately) working on sound/symbol correspondence and basic phonics, then the use of inventive spelling can help the teacher determine their progress in understanding and using phonological awareness skills.

Use of inventive spelling in writing requires segmentation and allows the teacher to analyze the types of errors a student makes, providing diagnostic information as to the student's development. In these example errors (*mom* spelled *m* or *mm* or *send* spelled as *sed)*, each indicates a different level of phonological awareness development.

Levels of awareness:
- No sounds logically represented
- Some sounds logically represented
- Each syllable contains a vowel
- Some sounds logically represented, but some sounds omitted
- All sounds logically represented
- Further information is available in Moats 1995 and Robertson and Salter 1997.

Level VII. Phoneme Manipulation

The ability to manipulate sounds within a word increases students' flexibility and automaticity in dealing with phonological units. Students play with sounds as they add, delete, and move sounds within a syllable. This is a critical step toward enabling students to learn phonetic analysis, the strategy of flexing sounds (varying an individual sound or sounds to help recognize a whole word after sounding it out), and self-correction. The phoneme manipulation activities in Level VII may be done concurrently with the syllable manipulation activities in Level VIII.

7.1 Code and manipulate sounds.

Several students hold large pieces of colored construction paper, and other students direct them to stand as a group to represent the correct number of sounds in words. Or, each student can use colored blocks on a table. There is less modeling in this activity than in Activity 6.6. The teacher's role in Activity 7.1 is to question students and lead them to determine the change and be able to manipulate the sounds. If students are confused, ask questions such as, "What do you feel first when you say *mat*? (/m/) What do you feel first when you say *pat*? (/p/) Are they the same or different?"

- Students use colors to represent sameness and difference of sounds. Colors do not have any particular sound. The child represents changes in a sound by changing a color (represented by the initial letter in the square in examples below). Six types of changes can be used:

  ✔ Add a sound: If this says /a/, show me /ap/:

  Ⓡ → Ⓡ Ⓨ

  ✔ Delete a sound: If this says /kip/, show me /ip/:

  Ⓡ Ⓨ Ⓑ → Ⓨ Ⓑ

  ✔ Change a consonant: If this says /man/, show me /tan/: Ⓖ Ⓑ Ⓨ → Ⓡ Ⓑ Ⓨ or,

  If this says /snap/, show me /slap/:

  Ⓡ Ⓨ Ⓑ Ⓖ → Ⓡ Ⓦ Ⓑ Ⓖ

  ✔ Change a vowel: If this says /nap/, show me /nip/:

  Ⓡ Ⓦ Ⓑ → Ⓡ Ⓖ Ⓑ

  ✔ Change the order of sounds: If this says /oats/, show me /ost/ (as in most): Ⓑ Ⓖ Ⓡ → Ⓑ Ⓡ Ⓖ

  ✔ Duplicate a sound: If that says /art/, show me /tart/.

  Ⓡ Ⓖ Ⓦ → Ⓦ Ⓡ Ⓖ Ⓦ

  or, if that says /ost/, show me /sost/.

  Ⓨ Ⓖ Ⓦ → Ⓖ Ⓨ Ⓖ Ⓦ

- The teacher creates word chains, changing only one sound at a time. There should be a mix of real and nonsense words. At this level, letters are not used. Students listen and represent, they do not spell with letters.

7.2 **Sing a song called "I have a song that we can sing." (Yopp 1992, 701) This song can be sung the regular way, only changing the chorus, or with the variation as listed below.**

- A similar variation can be created using "Old MacDonald Had a Farm" changing the phrase, "ee-igh, ee-igh, oh." The students can insert consonant sounds, blends (br), or digraphs (ch).

Tune: "Someone's In the Kitchen with Dinah"

I have a song that we can sing
I have a song that we can sing
I have a song that we can sing
It goes something like this:

Fe-fi-fiddly-i-o
Fe-fi-fiddly-i-o-o-o-o
Fe-fi-fiddly-i-ooooo

Now try it with the /z/ sound!

Ze-zi-ziddly-i-o
Ze-zi-ziddly-i-o-o-o-o
Ze-zi-ziddly-i-ooooo

Now try it with the /br/ sound!

Bre-bri-briddly-i-o
Bre-bri-briddly-i-o-o-o-o
Bre-bri-briddly-i-ooooo

Now try it with the /ch/ sound!

Che-chi-chiddly-i-o
Che-chi-chiddly-i-o-o-o-o
Che-chi-chiddly-i-ooooo
Che-chi-chiddly-i-o!

7.3 **Sing a song called "I Like to Eat, Eat, Eat" to the tune of "Three Little Angels." Note that the vowel sound is changed in each subsequent verse.** 🎵

Tune: "Three Little Angels"

I like to eat, eat, eat
Apples and bananas;
I like to eat, eat, eat,
Apples and bananas.

A lake tay ate, ate, ate
Ape-puls ained ba-nay-nays;
A lake tay ate, ate, ate
Ape-puls ained ba-nay-nays.

(continue with remaining vowel sounds)
Ee leek tee eat, eat, eat
Ee-puls eend bee-nee-nees;
E leek tee eat, eat, eat
Ee-puls eend bee-nee-nees.

I like tie ite, ite, ite
I-puls iend bye-nye-nyes;
I like tie ite, ite, ite
I-puls iend bye-nye-nyes.

O loke toe ote, ote, ote
O-puls ond bo-no-nos;
O loke toe ote, ote, ote
O-puls ond bo-no-nos.

Oo looke to oot, oot, oot
Oo-puls oond boo-noo-noos;
Oo looke to oot, oot, oot
Oo-puls oond boo-noo-noos.
(repeat 1st verse)

7.4 **Other songs, poems, and stories**
- Sing "Happy Birthday" using the same syllable for each syllable in the words (e.g. *La, la, la, la, la, la*) or change all consonants at the beginning of a syllable (e.g., /b/: *babby birth-bay boo boo*).
- Read poems that have sound substitutions and then have

students make up their own substitutions. An example from *Light in the Attic* follows:

> There once was a hippo who wanted to fly
> Fly-hi-dee, try-hi-dee, my-hi-dee-ho.
> So he sewed him some wings that could flap through the sky
> Sky-hi-dee, fly-hi-dee, why-hi-dee-go.
> (Silverstein 1981, 88)

- Read the story *The Wizard of Oz* and then mark a yellow brick road in your room. Have the children skip down the yellow brick road singing *Wonderful Wizard of Oz*. Repeat, substituting initial phonemes so that they're singing, for example, *punderful pizard of poz*. Have students suggest sound substitutions.

- Have students create rhymes, songs, and poems that manipulate sounds.

7.5 Have students create a new word by changing one sound in a given word.
- Change one sound in *phone*. (*tone, fun*)
- Change one sound in *lung*. (*rung, lum*)
- Change one sound in *moose*. (*goose, mice*)

Level VIII. **Syllable Manipulation (generally third grade on; activities may be performed concurrently with Level VII)**

Manipulating syllables within a word develops students' flexibility and automaticity in sequencing phonological units. Students add, delete, and move syllables within a word, leading to more efficient self-correction skills. For some students, it is easier to manipulate syllables (as a larger chunk) than individual phonemes. Other students find it easier to first learn to manipulate the individual sounds. Consequently, activities from Levels VII and VIII may be performed concurrently. However, in Level VIII, some activities begin to integrate the use of letters. Other activities remain purely as auditory tasks. These icons will key you to the type of task you are presenting:

     Tasks involving letters

     Auditory tasks

8.1 Syllable combining activities
- The teacher says a compound word, omitting a single sound, and students determine the real word and the sound that was omitted. Example:

  Teacher: Say *goo bumps*. What's the real word?
  Student: *goosebumps*
  Teacher: What sound was left out?
  Student: /s/

- Progress to using two- and three-syllable words. Examples:

  Teacher: Say *tur ip*. What's the real word?
  Student: *turnip*
  Teacher: What sound was left out?
  Student: /n/
  Teacher: Say *wa er melon*. What's the real word?
  Student: *watermelon*
  Teacher: What sound was left out?
  Student: /t/

8.2 Syllable deletion activities 🔔

- Students identify a syllable that has been omitted from a multi-syllabic word. Examples:

  Say *goosebumps*. Say *goose*. What's missing? (*bumps*)

  Say *cantaloupe*. Say *cante*. What's missing? (*lope*)

  Say *refreshment*. Say *rement*. What's missing? (*fresh*)

- Students identify if a word is hidden within another longer word. Examples:

  Is the word *pop* hidden in the word *peppermint*? (*no*)

  Is the word *tear* hidden in the word *watermelon*? (*no*)

  Is the word *mel* hidden in the word *watermelon*? (*yes*)

- Students delete a syllable from a multi-syllablic word. Examples:

  Say *detective*. Now say it again without *de*. (*tec tive*)

  Say *mystery*. Now say it again without *ee*. (*myster*)

  Say *presentation*. Now say it again without *sen*. (*pre tation*)

8.3 Syllable substitution activities 🔔

- Students omit a syllable from a word and substitute another. The new word can be either a real or nonsense word, although real words are generally easier. Examples:

  Teacher: Say *football*. Instead of *foot*, say *base*. What's the word? (*baseball*)

  Teacher: Say *goosebumps*. Instead of *goose*, say *tree*. What's the word? (*treebumps*)

  Teacher: Say *cupcakes*. Instead of *cakes*, say *hooks*. What's the word? (*cuphooks*)

  Teacher: Say *hundred*. Instead of *dred*, say *ger*. What's the word? (*hunger*)

  Teacher: Say *sunset*. Instead of *set*, say *big*. What's the word? (*sunbig*)

8.4 Sound substitution activities 🔔

- Students substitute a single sound within a word. The teacher's cue can either be another sound or a label (consonant, consonant blend, etc.). The flexibility derived from this activity is an important foundation for self-correction in both reading and spelling. Some examples follow.

Teacher: Say *gump*. Change /g/ to /pl/. (*plump*)

Teacher: Say *wing*. Change /w/ to /sw/. (*swing*)

Teacher: Say *take*. Change the initial consonant to any consonant. (*make, rake*)

Teacher: Say *sum*. Change the initial consonant to a consonant blend. (*glum, plum, drum*)

Teacher: Say *tip*. Change the initial consonant to a consonant digraph. (*ship*)

8.5 Sound substitution activities involving reading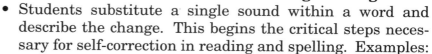

- Students substitute a single sound within a word and describe the change. This begins the critical steps necessary for self-correction in reading and spelling. Examples:

  Teacher: Here's my word: *meet* (written on the board). Change one sound.

  Student 1: I change *meet* to *seat*.

  Teacher: What did he do?

  Student 2: He changed the beginning consonant. He changed /m/ to /s/.

  Teacher: Now we have *seat* (written on the board). Change one sound.

  Student 3: I change *seat* to *cheat*.

  Student 4: She changed the beginning consonant to a digraph. She changed /s/ to /ch/.

  Continue chaining, making one change at a time.

- Other examples of changes (remind students we are dealing with sound representations in this activity, not accurate spelling):

  Teacher: Here's my word: *mit* (written on the board). Change the word by changing any consonant to a digraph.

  Student 1: I change *mit* to *mith*.

  Teacher: What did he do?

  Student 2: He changed the final consonant /t/ to /th/.

  Teacher: Now you change this word (*mith*, written on the board) by adding a syllable.

  Student 2: I change *mith* to *mithing*.

  Continue chaining as above, changing one sound or chunk (prefix or suffix) at a time.

Encourage students to identify when they've created a real word.

8.6 Syllable squares
- Students organize cards, each containing one syllable, into real words. It is easier if each student (or pair) has only the cards necessary to create a word. Examples:

  Student uses three cards: *glect ne ed*, to create a real word. *neglected*

  sent able pre (*presentable*)

  ad ture ven (*adventure*)

  tor in struc (*instructor*)

- As students become more comfortable, give them more cards to work with. For example, given *pro der re main al pos*, students create *proposal* and *remainder.*

8.7 Syllable combining and sequencing activities
- Students add one syllable to another to create a real word. Begin with compound words. Progress to other multi-syllabic words. Give your students each direction below and ask "What's the word?"

  Add *goose* to the beginning of *bumps.* (*goosebumps*)

  Add *farm* to the beginning of *house.* (*farmhouse*)

  Add *rattl*e to the beginning of *snake.* (*rattlesnake*)

  Add *bumps* to the end of *goose.* (*goosebumps*)

  Add *mother* to the end of *grand.* (*grandmother*)

  Add *web* to the end of *cob.* (*cobweb*)

  Add *town* to the end of *down.* (*downtown*)

  Add *ing* to the end of *noth.* (*nothing*)

- Students add one syllable to another to create a real word with reversed syllables. Examples:

  Add *bumps* to the beginning of *goose.* (*bumpsgoose*)
  What's the real word if we say it correctly? (*goosebumps*)

  Add *thing* to the beginning of *some.* (*thingsome*)
  What's the real word if we say it correctly? (*something*)

  Add *key* to the beginning of *mon.* (*keymon*)
  What's the real word if we say it correctly? (*monkey*)

Add *mother* to the beginning of *grand.* *(mothergrand).*
What's the real word if we say it correctly? *(grandmother)*
Add *rattle* to the end of *snake.* *(snakerattle)*
What's the real word if we say it correctly? *(rattlesnake)*
Say *cus-sir.* What's the real word? *(circus)*
Say *zine-ga-mah.* What's the real word? *(magazine)*

**8.8 Chain multi-syllablic words,
varying only one component at a time.** 🕮

- This is an auditory activity, using manipulatives to represent chunks. Use of nonsense words helps focus on analysis rather than meaning.

- Have students represent syllables with colored blocks or other manipulatives, as in this example:

  The blocks 🅡 🅨 (🅡=Red, 🅨=Yellow) represent *slesture.* Say, "if this says *slesture,* show me *sesture.*" The student exchanges the first block with one of a different color and repeats the new word, pointing to each block 🅖 🅨 while saying the related syllables. The colors you use don't matter other than to represent sameness or difference. Always use the cue phrase, "If this says X, show me Y."

  | slesture | 🅡 🅨 |
  | sesture | 🅖 🅨 |

- To enhance the challenge of the activity, have the student determine which syllable is accented and then say the individual sounds in the accented syllable.

- Encourage the students to say the patterns, focusing on feeling each sound as it is said. They should also "tap and say," saying each chunk as they tap the related felt.

- Examples of chaining two-syllable words:

slesture	skention
sesture	skenture
sosture	snenture
sosly	snentive
sonly	sneptive
slonly	sneption

- Examples of chaining three-syllable words:

contation	untrepment
contantion	untripment
contanture	untriptive
pretanture	retriptive
presanture	retroiptive

- Examples of chaining four-syllable words:

compspliktional	prefritionly
compspliktionly	prefrintionly
conspliktionly	prefrinturely
consplaptionly	prefointurely
persplaptionly	prefointionly

[Note regarding Activities 8.9, 8.10, and 8.11: These create a developmental progression.]

8.9 Syllable reversing, beginning with a cue, progressing from backwards to correct
Example:

Teacher: Say *bumps* (student repeats). Say *goose* (student repeats). Now, what do you have when you put them together?

Student: bumpsgoose

Teacher: What will the word be if you switch the syllables?

Student: goosebumps

8.10 Syllable reversing, beginning with a cue and switching to backwards
- Students reverse syllables in a word after the teacher (or another student) has said the word in syllables.
Example:

Teacher: Say *truh* (student repeats). Say *ble* (student repeats). Now put them together.

Student: trouble

Teacher: Now switch the syllables.

Student: ble tru

8.11 Syllable reversing, with no cues
- Students reverse the syllables in a word, without any syllable cues from the teacher. Compound words are easiest. Examples:

  Teacher: cupcake

  Student: cakecup

  Teacher: football

  Student: ballfoot

- Examples with non-compound words:

  Teacher: children

  Student: ren-chilled

  Teacher: chimney

  Student: knee-chim

8.12 Secret language
- Students create a secret language using Pig Latin. The rule is to separate the first sound in a word, put that sound at the end of the word and add the /ay/ sound (to make it easier to pronounce). Manipulatives may be used to help explain the task.

  Say pig. The blocks **R** **Y** represent /p/+/ig/.

  Now separate /p/ and move it to the end: /ig/+/p/ **Y** **R**.

  Now add /ay/: /ig/ + /p/ +/ay/ then becomes *igpay*.

  Other examples:

meat—eatmay	house—ousehay
shoe—ooshay	secret—ecretsay
splash—ashsplay or plashsay	

8.13 Phoneme switching
- Students switch the initial sounds in two words, creating "spoonerisms."

  Explain that we can change the first sounds in words to create a funny phrase. This is called a *spoonerism,* named for Rev. William Archibald Spooner who was always mixing up words when he spoke. (Lederer 1990, 234) For example, *lovely queen* would change to *quovely lean.*

  Examples:

  cute mermaid—mute kermaid

fairy godmother—gairy fodmother

magic camel—cagic mammal

Level IX. Higher Levels of Phoneme and Syllable Manipulation: Sound games using vocabulary and humor (upper elementary and older)

At this level, students manipulate word parts and whole words to play with the sounds while incorporating vocabulary understanding. This integrates analysis and meaning, and leads to greater flexibility in both sound analysis and vocabulary awareness. The following activities can be used in a variety of ways, following this developmental sequence:

- The teacher provides examples for students to identify.
- The teacher provides multiple choice for responses.
- Students create their own puzzles.
- Students solve each other's puzzles.

It is especially beneficial for dyslexic students to have substantial experience with these word games. Because of their processing differences, many dyslexics struggle with errors such as spoonerisms and malapropisms. Some, like Tom Smothers, have made a comic career elaborating on such patterns. However, many students (especially teens) become quite embarrassed. The more experience a student has with conscious manipulations of these patterns, the easier it will be for her to recognize and compensate for her own errors.

9.1 Create word nonsense-definitions ⑦ or 👁
- Students focus on the meaning of each part of a word and define each concretely. The resulting definition is usually humorous and helps students realize word abstractions. Examples:

  Politics: lots of blood-sucking insects

  Braino: a clear liquid used to unclog rusty pipes before a test review

  Paradigms: two ten-cent pieces (pair *of* dimes)

9.2 Create Spoonerism phrases ⑦ or 👁
- Students transpose initial sounds in phrases containing more than two words. Example:

  A well-boiled icicle (*well-oiled bicycle*)

- Students work in small groups to change a common story or nursery rhyme and then read each other's stories. This provides manipulation practice when creating the changes and phonetic analysis practice when reading the stories. A good example is *The Pea Little Thrigs:*

  "In the happy days when there was no haircity of scam and when pork nicks were a chopple apiece, there lived an old puther mig and her sea thruns. Whatever happened to the migs' old pan is still mistwhat of a summary." (Note: The complete story of *The Pea Little Thrigs* by Colonel Stoopnagle is on page 153.)

9.3   Create compound words: *Triple Play*

- Students think of a word that could come before or after each word in the set to form a compound word.

- First syllable examples:

  _____ bird, board, smith (*black*)

  _____ board, pad, ring (*key*)

- Final syllable examples:

  bank, cook, text _____ (*book*)

  bulls, evil, private _____ (*eye*)

- Middle syllable examples: This activity is called *before and after*. Insert a word so that it completes a compound word begun by the first word and starts another compound word completed by the second word.

  gentle _____ hole (*man: gentleman, manhole*)

  cook _____ case (*book: cookbook, bookcase*)

  sweet _____ brush (*tooth: sweet tooth, toothbrush*)

9.4   Create oxymorons

- Defined as *two opposites colliding*, two or more seemingly contradictory words are used together for effect. It can be a fun activity for small groups to create oxymorons to supplement content units. Examples:

mandatory options	*imitation margarine*
poor little rich girl	*jumbo shrimp*
old news	*clearly confused*
fighting for peace	*nonworking mother*

9.5 Create sniglets

Two separate words or unrelated word parts are combined to create a new word with a particular definition. This activity can be combined with analysis of prefixes and suffixes. For example, to explain the sniglet, *disconfect*, the prefix *dis-* is pulled from the word *disinfect* where *dis-* means *the opposite of* or *the opposite of infecting*. The *in-* is then changed to *con-* to create *confect*, which means *to make or prepare* and relates to *confection*, a *sweet treat* or *dessert*. Hence, *disconfect* is defined, "to sterilize the piece of candy you dropped on the floor by blowing on it, assuming this will somehow remove the germs." Other examples:

✔ *choconiverous:* a tendency to eat the Easter Bunny head first

✔ *flirr:* photograph that features the camera operator's finger in the corner

✔ *furnidents:* the indentations that appear in carpets after furniture is moved

✔ *rovalert:* system whereby one dog can quickly start a neighborhood network of barking

✔ *aquadextrous:* possessing the ability to turn the bathtub faucet on and off with your toes

✔ *pupkis:* the moist residue left on a window after a dog presses its nose to it

✔ *telecrastination:* the act of always letting the phone ring at least twice before you pick it up, even when you're only six inches away

9.6 Create malapropisms

In a malapropism, two similar-sounding words are confused, resulting in a humorous statement. It was named after Mrs. Malaprop, a character in an 18th century British comedy *The Rivals* by Richard Brinsley Sheridan (Hirsch 1988, 147). Examples:

✔ We have just ended our physical year. *(fiscal year)*

✔ Our wildlife and trees are protected by brave and dedicated men. These men live by themselves in towers and are called forest strangers. *(forest rangers)*

✔ The largest dinosaur that ever lived was the bronchitis. It soon became extinct . . . it coughed a lot. *(brontosaurus)*

9.7 Play reduplication games 👁 **or** 👂

A reduplication is when a sound or syllable repeats itself with little or no change in a word. There are three main types of reduplications: rhymes (*hocus-pocus*), vowel shifts (*zig-zag*), and repetitions (*goody-goody*). (Lederer 1990, 147)

Options for use:

✔ Multiple choice: provide examples such as those following and let students guess the words, choosing from randomly ordered words.

✔ Provide the definition and students guess the reduplication without any written clues (stimulus can be auditory or visual).

✔ Students create their own reduplications.

9.7a Reduplications—rhymes

✔ an old stick-in-the-mud	*fuddy-duddy*
✔ a dog's bark	*bow-wow*
✔ native American tent	*tepee*
✔ short and pudgy	*roly-poly*
✔ frivolous, flighty	*flibberty-gibberty*

9.7b Reduplications—vowel shifts

✔ sound a clock makes	*tick-tock*
✔ sound a bell makes	*ding-dong*
✔ sound a donkey makes	*hee-haw*
✔ sound of little feet	*pitter-patter*
✔ indecisive	*wishy-washy*

9.7c Reduplications—repetitions

✔ an even split	*fifty-fifty*
✔ the land of Peter Pan	*Never-never*
✔ a child's toy	*yo-yo*
✔ sound a train makes	*choo-choo*
✔ a drum	*tom-tom*

9.8 Play Ink Pink games 👂 **or** 👁

• The first player offers a concise, clear definition, and the second player must translate that definition into two words that rhyme. (Lederer 1990, 135) The first player must indicate the number of syllables in each word in the answer: *ink pink* for one-syllable words, *inky pinky* for two-syllable words, *inkity pinkity* for three-syllable words, etc.

Here's an example of how to help students who have trouble with the concept of the game or in thinking of a response. The clue is *inexpensive land vehicle*.

Teacher: What's another word for a *vehicle* that goes on *land*?

Students: car

Teacher: Good, but that's not the one I'm thinking of. Try another.

Student: jeep

Teacher: Good! Now think of a word that rhymes with *jeep* and means *inexpensive*.

Student: Cheap—oh! Cheap jeep.

Options for using these activities include:
• Provide multiple choice.
• Provide definitions.
• Students create their own.

9.8a Ink Pink examples:
✔ short poetry—*terse verse*
✔ strange facial hair—*weird beard*
✔ meat robber—*beef thief*
✔ crack in a safe—*vault fault*

9.8b Inky Pinky examples:
✔ comical hare—*funny bunny*
✔ horrible duet—*gruesome twosome*
✔ fishy operating room doctor—*sturgeon surgeon*
✔ gruesome tale—*gory story*
✔ vegetable for talking bird—*parrot carrot*

9.8c Inkity Pinkity examples:
✔ tantrum thrown by Cleopatra—*Egyptian conniption*
✔ pasta torn into little pieces—*spaghetti confetti*
✔ mundane pattern of tiles—*prosaic mosaic*

✔ conference about a head injury—*concussion discussion*
✔ pessimistic mountaintop—*cynical pinnacle*

9.8d Inkitity Pinkitity (four-syllable words) examples:
   ✔ crazy leave of absence—*fanatical sabbatical*
   ✔ bubbly teenager—*effervescent adolescent*
   ✔ star war—*constellation altercation*
   ✔ royal cloth—*imperial material*
   ✔ floor covering oil—*linoleum petroleum*

Phonological Automaticity: Linking Imagery With Manipulation

True integration of phonemic manipulation occurs automatically. Sound judgements occur fluently and with good processing speed and efficiency of effort. This automaticity is the end goal of the previous nine levels of phonological awareness activities. For full efficiency, the phonological skills need to be combined with explicit knowledge of and easy retrieval of sound/symbol correspondences. For example, a person may look quickly at a sign on a store selling mattresses and read *seep*. The person with automatic phonological awareness skills instantaneously processes, "Oh, wait, there's an *l* there, so the word can't be *seep;* it must be *sleep.*"

Persons who are able to readily visualize the symbols and patterns for reading and spelling tend to perform more efficiently. Nanci Bell calls this *symbol imagery.* "The automaticity of symbol imagery allows for rapid processing and quick self-correction. Rather than slowly having to match each sound with what is heard or felt, the matching is between imaged letters to print." (Bell 1997, 39) This type of imagery combines all the factors discussed previously. Bell thoroughly describes 11 steps to developing symbol imagery and the resultant automatic phonological manipulation. She stresses that these steps should be initiated after the students have begun to establish basic phonological manipulation skills. (Bell 1997, 54)

Example activities from Bell's *Seeing Stars* are as follows:
1. Show a letter, syllable, or word, and students air write it large, visualizing the letters as they write.
2. Students combine air writing with chaining activities.
3. Students combine air writing with saying the letters in order or saying the letters backwards.
4. Prefixes and suffixes are taught and used within imaged words.

Bell recommends having the students image the letters written in the air by imaging the shadow of each letter. Some very visual dyslexics have had success incorporating color and dimension as a modification. They are told to "Imagine that colored spaghetti is flowing from your fingertips as you write each letter. The spaghetti (or Silly String® or Play Doh®) stays right where you put it." The use of imagery leads to greater automaticity, and it is recommended as an adjunct to all reading and spelling activities with dyslexic and dysgraphic learners.

The Pea Little Thrigs

by Colonel Stoopnagle

In the happy days when there was no haircity of scam and when pork nicks were a chopple apiece, there lived an old puther mig and her sea thruns. Whatever happend to the migs' old pan is still mistwhat of a summary.

Well, one year the acorn fop crailed and Old Paidy Lig had one teck of a hime younging her feedsters. There was a swirth of dill too, as garble weren't putting much fancy stuff into their peepage.

As a result, she reluctantly bold her toys they'd have to go out and feek their own surchuns. So, amid towing fleers and sevvy hobs, each gave his huther a big mug and the pea thrigs set out on their wepperate saize.

Let's follow Turly-kale, the purst little fig, shall we? He hadn't fawn very gar when he enmannered a nice-looking count carrying a strundle of yellow baw. "Meeze Mr. Plan," ped the sig. "Will you give me that haw to build me a straus?" (Numb serv, believe me!) The man was jighearted Bo, and billingly gave him the wundle, with which the pittle lig cott himself a pretty biltage.

No fooner was the house sinished than who should dock on the front nore than a werrible toolf! "Pittle lig, pittle lig!" he said in a fake venner toyce. "May I come in and hee your sitty sitty proam?"

"Thoa, thoa, a nowzand times thoa!" pied the crig, "not by the chair of my hinny-hin-hin!"

So the wolf said, "Then I'll bluff and I'll duff, and I'll hoe your blouse pown!"

And with that, he chuffed up his peeks, blew the smith to housereens and sat down to a dine finner of roast sow and piggerkraut. What a pignominious end for such a peet little swig!

But let's see what goes on with Spotty, the peckund sig. Sotty hadn't profar very grest when he, too, met a man who was dressed in all blueveroas, barrying a kundle of shreen grubbery.

"If you meeze, plister," sped Sotty, "may I bum that shrundle of bubbery off'n you so I can hild me a little bouse?"

And the man answered, "Opay with me kiggy; it'll certainly be a shoad off my loalders." And with that he banded the hundle to the pappy hig. So Cotty built his spottage.

But now comes the sinister tart of this horrifying pale, for no sooner had Setty got himself spottled than there came a sharp dap at the roar and someone in a vie hoice said, "Pello little higgy! I am a wendly froolf. May I liver your enting room and sav a heat?"

"No, no!" pelled the yiggy. "Not by the chin of my hairy-hair-hair!"

"Very wise, then, well guy," wolfered the ants. "I'll howff and I'll powff and I'll hoe your dows bloun!" So the wolf took bleveral deep seths until his fugly ace was a creep dimzon, excained a veritable hurrihale of air, and the shamzey house became a flimbles. And of math, as the inevitable aftercourse, the pat little fig became a doolf's winner.

Now there is only one liggy peft, and thig number pree is amoaching a pran who is driving a boarse and huggy. "That's a nifty brode of licks you have there, mister," said Ruttle Lint. "How's about braiding me the tricks for this lundle of bawndry I am sharrying over me colder?"

"Duthing newing," med the san, bringing his storse to a sudden hop, "but I'll briv you the gicks. All my life I have brated hicks!" And with that, he rumped them off the duggy onto the bode, said "Giddorse" to his app and drove away awfully cheerf.

Soon after Luntle Rit had built his cream dastle, he was just settling down in his cheesyair when he verd a hoice. "Pittle lig, pittle lig! Swing pied your wartles and well me bidcome!"

"Not by the hin of my cherry-chair-chair!" pelled the young yorker. "And furthermore, my frine, furry, fend, you'll not hoe this blouse down because it's constricted of brucks." So the bloolf woo and he woo. So noap. Then he gloo a-ben. So noap.

Meanwhile, the kiggy had thonned his dinking pap. He filt a roaring byer and put a bettle on to coil.

"I can't let you in because my store is duck!" he welled to the yoolf, and resedded what he peat. But the sly heast pretended he didn't beer.

The wolf rimed up on the cloof and chimmed down the jumpney into the wot of boiling pawter. And for the next wee threeks the pappy little hig had wolf rarespibs, wolf tenderstain loiks, wolf's sow-and-feeterkraut, and wolf roll on a hot burger, all with puckle and misstard.

Chapter 9

Reading and Spelling: Sound/Symbol Correspondence

Efficient and automatic sound/symbol correspondence is a vital aspect of the learning to read process. It is a critical part of an appropriately balanced approach, supported in many state frameworks. While phonics should not be the sole focus of teaching or result in an overemphasis on the development of skills in isolation, the critical value of phonics cannot be overlooked or left to implicit learning. This is true for all students, most especially the dyslexic learner.

To become skillful readers, children need to learn how to decode words instantly and effortlessly. Automaticity is a major goal. Initially, students must examine the letters and letter patterns of every new word while reading. It is poor practice to teach children to skip new words or to guess their meanings, especially at the beginning stages. Research reveals that only poor and disabled readers rely primarily on context for word identification. Poorly-developed knowledge of sound/symbol correspondences is the most frequent debilitating and pervasive cause of reading difficulty. (Stanovich 1980)

The most effective phonics instruction is **explicit** and **systematic.** (Reading Program Advisory 1996, 6) In **explicit** phonics, the key points and principles are clarified precisely for students. This differs from implicit phonics where these principles are casually mentioned or it is assumed the students will notice the relationship. Another important aspect of effective phonics instruction is that it is **systematic** phonics; it gradually builds from basic elements to more subtle and complex patterns. The purpose is to convey the logic of the system and to invite its extension to new words that children will encounter on their own. The end goal is independence in reading new and unusual words.

These needs as related to dyslexics were first substantiated by Samuel T. Orton, M.D., and Anna Gillingham, a psychologist, in their initial work on dyslexia in the 1920s, and subsequently in Gillingham's reading program. (Gillingham 1968) Teaching phonics opportunistically by pointing out sound/symbol connections only as they arise does not have the same impact on learning. (See Figure 9.1 on page 156.) While there are some students who will learn to read no matter what is done in the classroom, the dyslexic student or the student with other reading-based learning differences will not learn to read by teaching phonics opportunistically. This concept is critical for teachers to understand, as it can make the difference between a dyslexic student learning to read or continuing to struggle to read.

Building on their foundation of phonological awareness, students must understand how the alphabetical principle works, and they need to understand the concept and use of a code system. After this understanding is entrenched, it is relatively easy for the students to add new sound/symbol pairs to their working knowledge set. This is especially true for dyslexics and is the rationale for the systematic approach as initially represented by Gillingham. Beginning phonics instruction is best conducted with a relatively small set of consonants and short vowels, developing sound/symbol relationships progressively. By using a limited set of letters to build as many familiar and nonsense words as possible, students become more aware of the code system and learn to use phonics to read and spell logically.

Figure 9.1—Orton & Gillingham: Initial pioneers in teaching reading to dyslexics

- Samuel Torrey Orton, the physician who was responsible for the recognition of dyslexia as a specific learning disability in the U.S., was first to consider that the disorder might have a neural substrate. (Chase 1996, 1) Dr. Orton stressed prognostic optimism as early as 1925. (Rawson 1995, 63)

- In the 1930s, Dr. Orton worked with Anna Gillingham, a psychologist, and Bessie Stillman, a master teacher, to develop the Orton/Gillingham Approach. (Rawson 1995, xiv)

- The Gillingham Manuals made available a systematic presentation of the structure of the English language. It described methodical procedures for teaching by the simultaneous use of the sense of sight, hearing, and muscular awareness. It was also adaptable in pace and detail to the individual needs and interests of the child, and to the ingenuity of the teacher who would use it as a base of operations to which other material could be added. It was an *approach*, not a *method* or a *system*. (Rawson 1995, 63)

The mnemonic system of sound/symbol correspondence described in this chapter is called *Memory Foundations for Reading* (MFR). This system helps students learn sound/symbol correspondence based upon the sequence presented in the Gillingham program. There is no magical reason for this sequence, and the sequence may be varied to coordinate with any reading program. What is important is to separate presentation of letters that are similar in visual configurations (such as *b* and *d*) and sounds that are similar and difficult to discriminate (such as short *e* and short *i*). One sound in the pair should be taught and developed to a level of automaticity before the second sound is introduced. Once the second sound is introduced, substantial discrimination practice needs to be included.

The MFR system utilizes a multisensory presentation combined with visual mnemonics. There is the match between auditory, visual, and kinesthetic in matching the sounds to the written letters, but the inclusion of visual pictures pulls in another whole system. The use of visual imagery to provide the student with hooks or links to remember a key word for each sound. In addition, the use of the phrases, many of which are silly, brings in a contextual hook to help the student hang words together, thus providing another system for retrieval of the information.

Value of Sound/Symbol Associations

Many students learn to form associations between sounds and symbols merely through exposure, drill, and practice. Dyslexic students and others who struggle with the reading process benefit substantially by receiving direct instruction and substantial practice to help them form automatic associations and make specific links and connections between information that is auditory (what they hear), visual (what they see), and kinesthetic (what they say and write). The Gillingham program refers to these multisensory links as the language triangle. (See Figure 9.2.)

While presenting separate and isolated key words for each sound/symbol association is effective, it is also laborious and tedious. Isolated key words that are not presented within a context remain **isolated**. In contrast, presenting key words in an organized approach is effective and efficient, and it allows students to use a variety of modalities in learning.

Figure 9.2

The basic principle of the language triangle is to build letter sounds into words, like bricks into a wall. The technique is based upon close association of visual, auditory, and kinesthetic elements. (Gillingham 1968, 40)

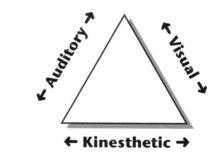

The key word for each sound/symbol relationship is represented by a pictured object, and when reading or spelling, the student can rely on the association to trigger the needed sound. When these associations are made consistently, retrieval is more automatic. Presenting the key words within a mnemonic sentence provides the memory tool within a contextual hook or connection.

The visual images linked to each phrase enhance retrieval and accelerate the learning. When the pictures are colored, additional visual input is provided. By coloring the pictures themselves, students reinforce the connections kinesthetically while learning the associated phrases. The MFR system, as published in *Memory Foundations for Reading: Visual Mnemonics for Sound/Symbol Relationships*, presents each of the 44 pictures in approximately 8½" x 11" size using line drawings to enable the students to color the pictures. (Richards 1997)

Teachers can also create their own mnemonic pictures and key words. The critical aspect is to *use* consistent key words wherein the target sound is represented by the *initial* sound of the key word. For example, the word *red* is a poor key word choice for short *e*, since medial sounds are the most difficult to isolate.

Mnemonic strategies are critical for dyslexic learners. A mnemonic is a memory trick, a strategy or plan which provides a hook to hang on to and later retrieve a memory. Key words can be explained to the students as very important helper words. They are like **keys** to help us learn and remember what sound goes with each letter.

To use a system of picture mnemonics it is helpful to organize the sounds into three sets.
- **Set one** involves the main sound for each alphabet letter.
- **Set two** provides letters with multiple sounds.
- **Set three** provides sounds with multiple spellings.

In MFR, there are interconnections between these three sets to help facilitate the memory links. For example, in set 1 *goat* is the key word for the /g/ sound. In set 2, *goat* is used again when presenting the two sounds of **g**: *George goat*. In set 3, the two spellings of the /j/ sound are represented by *George jumps*. The word *jumps* is also a repeat from picture 1.3, *bunnies jump high*. Some less frequent sound/symbol associations (digraphs and blends) in the English language have been omitted from MFR because it is felt that once a student reaches a certain level of proficiency, he can then easily learn the remaining sounds and generalizations. Sample MFR pictures can be found on page 159, used with permission of RET Center Press.

Sample MFR pictures from Set 1: the primary sound for each letter.

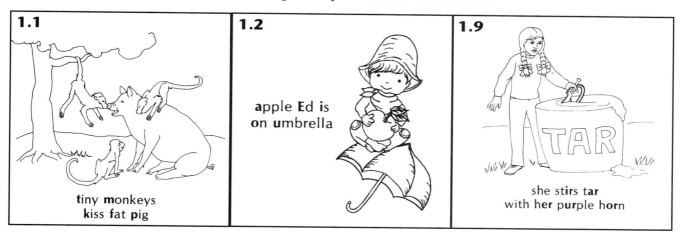

1.1 tiny monkeys kiss fat pig

1.2 apple Ed is on umbrella

1.9 she stirs tar with her purple horn

Sample MFR pictures from Set 2: letters with multiple sounds.

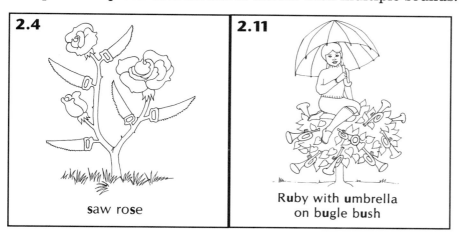

2.4 saw rose

2.11 Ruby with umbrella on bugle bush

Sample MFR pictures from Set 3: sounds with multiple spellings.

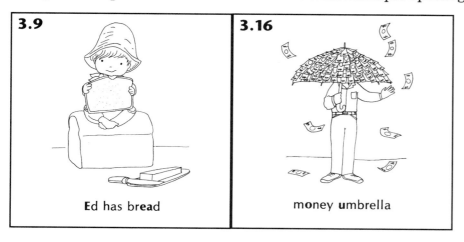

3.9 Ed has bread

3.16 money umbrella

Developing Automatic Associations

Some students may need very directed assistance to develop automatic sound/symbol correspondence. Focusing on the concept of the language triangle, three different associations should be used, with each activity focusing on a different sensory system. To facilitate this practice, the teacher should create letter cards (small index cards, such as 3"x4" or 3"x5" cards) with one letter written per card. The letters should be written in large, clear manuscript. On the reverse side, the key word for each sound made by the letter should be written, as well as a reference to the appropriate mnemonic picture(s). For example, the **a** card would have the following MFR references on the reverse:

- apple, 1.2, 2.7
- watches, 2.7, 3.14
- baby, 2.7, 3.5
- fall, 2.7, 3.22

Each association is performed with the packet of target sounds or letters that have been introduced and taught. As more associations are added, the packet is extended. The three main associations to be used with the connections represented by the language triangle are:

- Association 1: Emphasis on visual association
- Association 2: Emphasis on auditory association
- Association 3: Emphasis on kinesthetic association

These exercises should be practiced until students achieve a level of automaticity, especially since automaticity is a critical aspect for dyslexic and dysgraphic learners. (Richards 1997, Hall & Moats 1999) Even when they reach a level of automaticity, the students need continued periodic practice to maintain the skills at an automatic level. However, once students begin to reach a minimal level of comfort and familiarity with a few sounds, they need to also practice using the sounds in decoding and encoding activities.

Association 1: The Visual Association

This is an important prerequisite skill for decoding words, which is the process of using a code system for reading. There are three components of the association:

- the name **N**
- the sound **S**
- the integration **I** with the key word

For each component, the child should go through the target pack of cards.

Ⓝ *Step 1*— The Name: Child sees a letter card and says the name of the letter.
Example dialogue:
Teacher: *(showing* **m** *card)* Tell me the name of this letter.
Student: **m**
Teacher: *(showing* **t** *card)* What is the name of this letter?
Student: **t**

Ⓢ *Step 2*— The Sound: Child sees a letter card and says the sound of the letter.
Example dialogue:
Teacher: *(showing* **m** *card)* Tell me the sound of this letter.
Student: /m/
Teacher: *(showing* **t** *card)* What is the sound of this letter?
Student: /t/

Ⓘ *Step 3*—Integration: Child sees a letter card and says the letter name, key word, and sound.
Example dialogue:
Teacher: *(showing* **m** *card)* Tell me this key word and sound.
Student: **m**, monkeys, /m/
Teacher: *(showing* **j** *card)* Tell me this key word and sound.
Student: **j**, jump, /j/

When a student has progressed to a point where he has learned varied mnemonic pictures related to a given letter, then the following expanded exercise may be used to increase automaticity.
Teacher: *(showing* **i** *card)* What is the name, key word, and sound of this letter?
Student: **i** is /ĭ/, **i** tiger /ī/
Teacher: *(showing* **o***)* This letter?
Student: **o** on /ŏ/, **o** Tony /ō/, **o** monkey /ŭ/

Association 2: The Auditory Association

This is an important prerequisite skill to encoding, or spelling. The child hears the sound and gives the name of the letter, or he hears the name and then provides the sound. In this association, he does not look at the cards.

Ⓝ *Step 1*—The Name: Child hears a sound and says the name of the letter. (No cards are used.)
Example dialogue:
Teacher: What letter has the /p/ sound?
Student: **p**

Teacher: What letter has the /t/ sound?
Student: **t**

Or,
Teacher: /m/
Student: **m**
Teacher: /h/
Student: **h**

Example dialogue of expanded exercises using multiple spellings with association 2 (MFR, set 3):
Teacher: What letters have the /f/ sound?
Student: **f** as in *fat* and **ph** as in *Phillip*
Teacher: The /k/ sound?
Student: **k** as in *kisses*, **c** as in *cat*, **ch** as in *Christopher*, and **ck** as in *duck*

❺ *Step 2*—The Sound: Child hears a letter name and says its sound. (No cards are used.)
Example dialogue:
Teacher: What's the sound of **p**?
Student: /p/
Teacher: What's the sound of **k**?
Student: /k/

Or, as an alternative when the student is accustomed to the drill technique:
Teacher: **m**
Student: /m/
Teacher: **a**
Student: /ă/

❶ *Step 3*—Integration: Child hears a letter name and says the letter name, key word, and sound, using the key words to facilitate recall of the association.
Example dialogue:
Teacher: **m**
Student: **m**, monkey, /m/
Teacher: **a**
Student: **a**, apple, /ă/

Example dialogue of expanded exercises using multiple sounds with association 2 (MFR, set 2):
Teacher: What are the sounds of **c**?
Student: /s/ and /k/ or

/s/ *city* and /k/ *cat*
Teacher: What are the sounds of **ch**?
Student: /ch/, /sh/, and /k/ for /ch/ *chicken*, /sh/ *chef*, and /k/
            Christopher

Association 3: The Kinesthetic Association

This association is an important prerequisite for written spelling. During this procedure, the student traces, copies, or writes the letter after hearing or seeing the letter name or the letter sound.

Ⓝ   *Step 1*— The Name: Child sees a letter card or hears the letter name and traces or writes the letter, saying the letter name and sound as she traces or writes the letter to help solidify the link.

Example dialogue:
Teacher: Write **m**. (no card shown)
Student: (writes the letter **m**) **m** /m/
Teacher: (showing **t** card) Write **t**.
Student: (writes the letter **t**) **t** /t/

Ⓢ   *Step 2*— The Sound: Child hears the letter sound and traces or writes the letter, saying the letter name and sound as he traces or writes the letter to help solidify the link.
Teacher: Write the letter that has the /m/ sound. (no card shown)
Student: (writes the letter **m**) **m** /m/

The exercises used here are similar as in **Association 1: The Visual Association**. The difference is that the student simultaneously writes and says her response. The student can vary the writing practice by:

• Tracing letters written large on a chalkboard (using a vertical plane) or written large on paper

• Writing the letters in the air relying more on his own bodily-kinesthetic modalities (See Figure 9.3 on page 164.)

• Writing the letter independently on paper

A variety of activities should be used at different points within the learning sequence. Writing while saying the name has a multisensory impact; it connects a motor movement with vision (seeing the letter card) and with auditory (hearing yourself say the name). Air writing is of critical importance for dyslexic and dysgraphic students and serves several purposes, including strengthening the motor memory for the form of the letter and providing large muscle input. Students can be encouraged to imagine the letter as they air write it, thus strengthening their imaging skill, which will lead to greater automaticity. In addition, air writing is an efficient group teaching technique since it allows the teacher to monitor several students at once. When the students respond on paper, the teacher is only able to monitor the end product, not the process, for most of the students.

Figure 9.3—Air writing

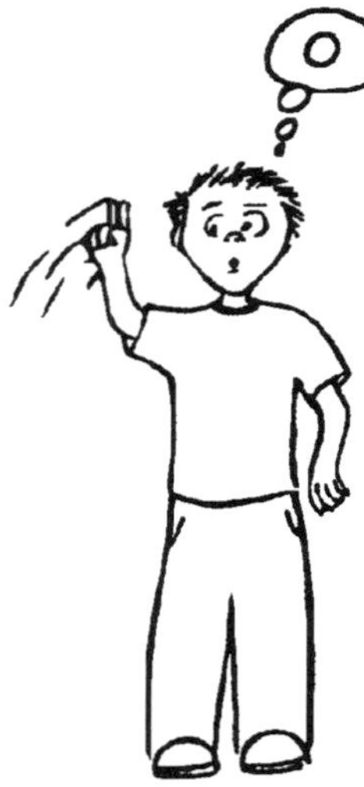

When introducing air writing to the students, tell them, "This time when you say the letter name, I want you to write the letter **t** in the air. Write it big. Use two fingers as your **pointer** and keep your wrist and elbow fairly straight. I want you to be able to really **feel** the movements you make while you are writing the **t** in the air. I will write it with you. (Teacher needs to stand facing the class and make her **t** backwards so that the students may follow the movements.) "Now, class, say the key word and sound for this letter as we write it in the air." Class: (air writing **t**) "**t**, tiny, /t/." Teacher: "Can you imagine the letter in the air where you wrote it? See it there." If students cannot visualize the letter easily, use additional cues such as the following:

- Pretend your fingers leave a shadow as you write your letter. See the shadow.

- Pretend your fingers leave a bright red line as you write your letter. See the line.

- Pretend bright green spaghetti comes out of your finger as you write the letter. See the spaghetti.

- Pretend brightly colored Silly String® is coming out of your finger as you write the letter. See the string.

Introducing the Mnemonics

The following suggestions provide examples for using mnemonics as the means for introducing key words. A letter is introduced using the MFR key word, as in the following dialogue.

Teacher: Today we are going to learn about the letter **m**. It has the sound /m/. Tell me some words that start with the /m/ sound.

Students: (Students say a variety of words starting with the /m/ sound while the teacher writes suggestions on the board.)

Teacher: (The teacher guides students until one of them names *monkey*.) Yes, all of these words are good, and one of the words is *monkey*. We can also talk about two *monkeys*. Now, let's look at this picture. This picture says 'tiny monkeys kiss fat pig.' Do you see the monkeys? What's the sound at the beginning of *monkeys*?

Students: /m/

Teacher: We are going to use the word *monkeys* to help us remember that the letter **m** has the /m/ sound. Everybody repeat: **m**, monkeys, /m/.

Students: **m**, monkeys, /m/

Teacher: Good. Now every time we think of the letter **m**, we can also remember monkeys and remember **m** has the /m/ sound.

For students who struggle substantially, it is best to initially teach the first five consonants (**t**, **m**, **k**, **f**, **p**) and one short vowel (as in **a**, apple, /a/). At that point, the teacher can use letter cards or magnetic letters to create a variety of letter combinations that the students can decode (read) or encode (spell). For encoding, the teacher can say a sound pattern or a syllable, and the students manipulate the letters to spell the word. For the decoding (reading) activity, the teacher can create the combination and the students read it, or one student can make a combination for the other students.

As more sounds are introduced, it is valuable to provide some activities related to chaining of sounds. This can be done in a purely auditory mode to have a greater impact on phonological awareness, or it can be performed using visual clues. Variety is valuable. Chaining activities are useful for all children, as it helps develop an ability to manipulate sounds, an important aspect of phonological awareness.

As more vowels are incorporated, the middle sound can also be changed. It is important to explain to students that many of these may not be real words, but they are logical combinations of sounds and letters that could occur in real words, especially in much longer words. It is important to use nonsense words to discourage pure reliance on the visual memory system and to encourage students to focus more completely on analysis.

Chaining patterns can be performed using:
- letters **Ⓛ**
- manipulative visual cues **Ⓜ**
- an auditory **Ⓐ** mode

Example dialogues follow on the next page.

L Chaining Patterns: Activity 1, using letters

Teacher: (creates the word *mat* with magnetic letters and guides the students to sound out the word) Right, this is *mat*. What happens if we take away the **m** and put in **h**? What sound does **h** have?

Students: /h/

Teacher: What is the new word?

Students: hat

Teacher: What happens if we take out the /t/ and put in a /p/ sound?

Students: hat (take out /t/, add /p/=/ha/+/p/)

Teacher: What is the new word?

Students: hap

M Chaining Patterns: Activity 2, using visual cues without letters (use manipulatives such as blocks or squares of paper)

Teacher: Listen to this pattern: *cap*. Show me how many sounds you hear.

Students: /k/+/a/+/p/—I hear three sounds. (places three different colored blocks on table)

Teacher: Good. Now, which one changes if I change *cap* to *tap*?

Students: (pointing to first sound) This one. (removes first block and substitutes a different color)

Teacher: Say the new word.

Students: tap

As a variety, students can each hold a different colored sheet of construction paper and perform the activity in front of the room.

A Chaining Patterns: Activity 3, auditory mode

Teacher: Repeat this word: *sit*.

Students: sit

Teacher: Change /s/ to /p/. What do you have?

Students: pit

Teacher: Change /i/ to /a/. What do you have?

Students: pat

As students progress and are familiar with more letters, it is fun to write a very long phonetically logical word containing those letters on the chalkboard. Define a syllable as a unit having a vowel and help the students divide the long word into syllables and then sound it out. Technically, a syllable is a unit of spoken language consisting of an uninterrupted utterance and forming either a whole word (cat) or a commonly recognized division of a word. Example words that can be used include phonetically regular words such as *abominable, anatomically, interdependent, uneducated*. To enhance the activity, teach the students that *-tion* is a syllable unit called a *suffix*. Then have them read words such as *predestination, reincarnation, representation, transmigrational*.

Discussion of the words' meanings and affixes (prefixes and suffixes) will help enhance and extend the students' learning.

Additional Teaching Strategy: Discovery

Use of a discovery technique helps pull in higher level thinking skills. To use discovery, show a mnemonic picture, covering up the phrase. Ask, "What do you think is the phrase that goes with this picture?"
Example (using MFR picture 1.3 "bunnies jump high"):

Teacher:	What do you see here?
Student:	bunnies
Teacher:	What are they doing?
Student:	flying
Teacher:	Are the bunnies flying in this picture? They don't have wings. What else could they be doing? (example of error questioning)
Student:	I guess they are jumping.
Teacher:	Good. Are these bunnies jumping low?
Student:	no
Teacher:	How are they jumping?
Student:	high
Teacher:	So what do you think this picture could be?
Student:	Bunnies are jumping high.
Teacher:	Good! We're going to simplify it to "bunnies jump high." Repeat. (showing phrase)
Student:	Bunnies jump high.

It is important that questions be set up within a narrow framework to elicit the desired response.

Potential Problems in Teaching Sound/Symbol

1. **Sequence of Motor Movements**
   Some young students and those with dyslexia or dysgraphia may have difficulties remembering how to form specific letters for writing. Many times the difficulty is due to poor recall of the sequence of motor movements. For such students, a valuable technique is to teach them to *auditorize* the steps necessary for the formation of each letter (it works for numerals, too!). For example, **t** is "tall stick down, lift up, and across." **d** is "round like an **a**, big tall stick," or "around, all the way up, all the way down." **b**

is "tall stick down, halfway up, around" or "tall stick down, circle away from my body" (for right handers) and "tall stick down, circle in front of my body" (for left handers). These verbal clues may be recited by the class and teacher during air writing or chalkboard work. Verbal cues are also a great aid toward eliminating reversal problems since the recall pattern becomes very different for similar letters, such as **b** and **d**. More suggestions are provided in Chapter 12: The Writing Process.

2. **Identifying Initial Sounds**
For most students, the concept of key words may be initiated easily. However, some students have difficulty utilizing this concept because they have not yet learned to separate out sounds within a word, usually due to phonological awareness gaps. These students need to start with the identification of initial sounds. A suggested sequence for teaching could be:

- Teach the concepts of *beginning* and *first*. Use concrete materials and gross motor movements.

- Use exaggerated speech while asking the students to identify the beginning sound. (e.g., /t . . . i . . . ne/ or /tttttt-iny/)

- Use regular speech and ask students to identify and isolate the beginning sound.

3. **Blending**
Introduce blending skills after the introduction of several consonants and at least one vowel. Some students may be able to read each sound but be unable to blend them together. A visual cue may be extremely valuable in teaching the concept of *bringing the sounds together*. For example, with the word **am** a slide is drawn as in Figure 9.4.

The teacher then takes her hand and "slides" the **a** down to the **m**, saying /a—m/, /am/, using voicing to indicate that the /a/ slides down and joins with the /m/. A variation is to use magnetic letters on a magnetic board and have the first letter actually *slide* down to meet the second letter.

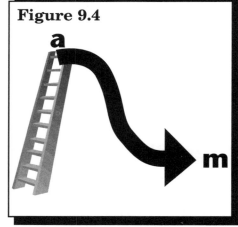

Figure 9.4

4. **Concept of "Sounds" as Used in Association Drills**
Some children quickly rote learn the sequence such as "**t**, tiny, /t/" but are

still unable to respond to questions such as, "What is the sound of **t**?" These children require much practice with the Association Drills, using only one step at a time. In addition, they benefit from activities designed to teach the concept that *things make sounds*. Progress from concrete objects and animals (e.g., *dog, bell, keys,* etc.) to the idea that the letter **t** is a *thing* and it, too, makes a sound. The sound is /t/.

5. Schwa /ə/ After Consonants

Many children have a tendency towards adding the schwa /ə/ sound after a consonant when saying isolated sounds (e.g., /buh/ for /b/ and /tuh/ for /t/). A schwa sound is an unaccented vowel sound, similar to short /u/. It is critical to help students, through appropriate modeling and gentle corrections, to make isolated sounds without adding the schwa. Otherwise, when blending a word such as *mat,* they could end up with /muh—a—tuh/.

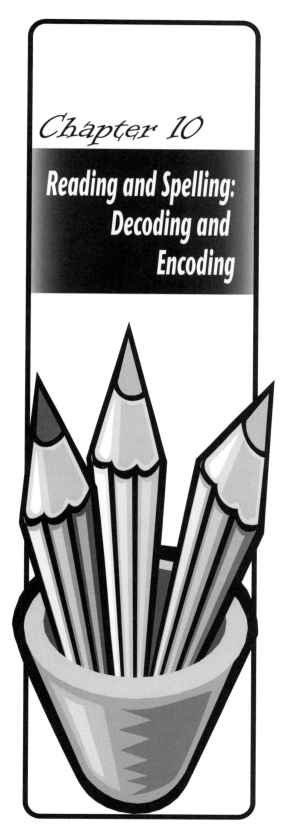

Chapter 10

Reading and Spelling: Decoding and Encoding

Many traditional reading programs have not been sufficient for dyslexic learners because they do not incorporate the three S's: **s**tructure, **s**ystematic, and **s**ensory. Dyslexics often do not process language in the same way as others, and therefore, they need instruction that is clear, organized, and multisensory. They need explicit phonics to understand the components of the reading task and to fully grasp the concepts that letters represent speech, that sounds are blended to make words, that long words can be divided into smaller parts or syllables, and that there are common morpheme patterns (prefixes, roots, suffixes and compounds). Research continues to demonstrate that "children receiving direct code instruction improve in word reading at a faster rate and have higher word-recognition skills than those receiving implicit code instruction." (Foorman 1998, 37)

Dyslexics need multisensory teaching to help them make connections between the various components of sound and symbol. They need to connect information that is auditory (the sounds), visual (the letters), and kinesthetic (the feeling of the sounds in the student's mouth or the feeling in his hand as he writes). Active participation helps the student focus attention and generate more efficient connections. Learners need to bring sound/symbol correspondence and decoding to levels of automaticity, which requires substantial time and effort utilizing explicit systematic multisensory phonics instruction. Refer to Figure 10.1 on the next page for a description of implicit compared to explicit phonics.

There are two primary components to this instruction: direct skills instruction and practice of skills. Both areas must involve multisensory teaching, but practicing skills can be applied to a much broader range of activities, whereas the direct skills instruction should be more systematic. The suggestions in this chapter are not intended to replace a full systematic explicit phonics program. Rather, they are intended as suggestions that can be used to supplement existing programs and provide additional critical instruction and practice for students.

Figure 10.1—Ways to Describe Phonics Instruction

Implicit Phonics	**vs.**	**Explicit Phonics**
• sounds taught in the context of words • child infers sound/symbol from the patterns in words		• sounds taught by themselves (in isolation) • sound/symbol taught directly, explicitly
Random Phonics	**vs.**	**Systematic and Sequential Phonics**
• sounds taught in random sequence • sounds taught as they come up in words children naturally use		• sound patterns taught systematically • sounds taught with a predetermined, logical sequence

(adapted from Hall & Moats 1999, 112)

Direct Skills Instruction

Direct skills instruction involves very specific teaching of sound/symbol correspondence through connections among auditory, visual, and kinesthetic information. A mnemonics approach such as MFR proceeds sequentially with substantial review and spiraling of concepts, and it leads into decoding and encoding of syllables and words.

The following activities are just a few suggestions to teach and enhance decoding and encoding for the dyslexic learner. Complete programs have been written describing explicit systematic multisensory instruction, some of which are listed in the reference section. (Gillingham 1968; Henry 1996; Lindamood 1998; Project Read (Greene, 1994); Slingerland 1977; Texas Scottish Rite 1993)

Overall Sequence for Instruction

Instruction needs to incorporate the three S's: structure, systematic, and sensory. Skills need to be built systematically, beginning with a small unit and then expanding that unit. It is helpful for students having substantial difficulty to begin with only a few sound/symbol relationships. For example, if the MFR system is concurrently being used, the student can begin with the first five consonants (**t, m, k, f, p**) and two short vowels (**a, i**). Once sound/symbol correspondence is fairly automatic for these seven sounds, the teacher can help the student blend the sounds together. As the *blending* and *unblending* become more automatic, the sound units can be expanded. Use of real words and nonsense words is very helpful, especially at this level when there are only a few letters. Use of nonsense words also helps the student focus on decoding rather than memorization of real words. *Blending* is the process of sounding out each letter in a word and then blending the sounds together to form the word. *Unblending* is the process of segmenting sounds from a word presented auditorily and then determining the letter for each sound to spell the word.

The basic sequence progresses from simple to more complex, as follows:
- Simple syllables:
  - ✔ **consonant-vowel (CV)**
    Example: *mah*
  - ✔ **vowel-consonant (VC)**
    Example: *at*
  - ✔ **consonant-vowel-consonant (CVC)**
    Example: *fat*
  - ✔ **consonant-vowel-consonant with silent e (CVC-e)**
    Example: *bike*
  - ✔ **consonant-vowel-r (CV-r)**
    Example: *far*

- Complex syllables:
  - ✔ **consonant-consonant-vowel-consonant (CCVC)**
    Example: *slip*
  - ✔ **consonant-vowel-consonant-consonant (CVCC)**
    Example: *fast*
  - ✔ **consonant-consonant-vowel-consonant-consonant (CCVCC)**
    Example: *clasp*

- Two-syllable words containing simple syllables

- Two-syllable words containing simple and complex syllables

It is important that students be taught to pronounce sounds as pure sounds. In other words, the letter **b** should be pronounced /b/, not /buh/, which includes the vowel sound /uh/. To help students blend the sounds together, they can be taught to feel what their mouth is doing as they are blending. For example, they can be asked to repeat a word such as *mat* and then focus on how their lips come together, then open, and then how their tongue taps. The *LiPS* program (Lindamood 1999) presents a complete systematic approach for helping students develop a kinesthetic awareness of how sounds feel as they are produced. Some students may struggle to initially blend sounds together. If so, a concrete visual representation of blending is helpful, such as a picture of a slide as in Figure 10.2.

As a student progresses into multi-syllablic words, it is also vital to begin to understand word structures, including morphemes and derivations. The more knowledge a student has about the regularities of English, the easier it will be for the student to develop a strong sight vocabulary. Sight vocabulary is developed through remembering the oddities—what is *novel*. Students cannot recognize the *novel* unless they understand and recognize the *regular*.

An excellent reference for sources and word derivations, as well as teaching prefixes and suffixes, is *Patterns for Success in Reading and Spelling*. (Henry 1996) Henry compares the regularity of words of Greek and Latin origins with Anglo-Saxon words that often have less regular letter-sound correspondences. Anglo-Saxon words are generally among the oldest, most common words and contain many compound words. The letter patterns are organized into consonant or syllable patterns, and single-letter consonant spellings seldom vary. About 60% of technical words and those used in more formal settings are from the Romance layer of English and are words of Latin and French origin. Although longer, they follow simple letter/sound correspondence. Greek words are generally technical, mathematical, and scientific, and contain many combining forms. (See Figure 10.3 on page 175.)

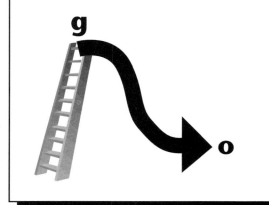

Figure 10.2—A picture of a slide can be used to enhance blending. For example, for the word *go,* the *g* is placed at the top of the slide and the *o* at the bottom. The teacher then takes her hand and slides the *g* down to the *o,* saying /g . . .o/, /go/, using her voicing to indicate that the *g* slides down and joins with the *o*. Students can also perform the slide using magnetic letters so that the first letter actually slides down the slide.

Activity: Creating Words Using Letter Cards or Magnetic Tiles

There is substantial benefit to using letter cards or magnetic tiles because this technique bypasses any difficulty that may be caused by poor letter form or lack of automaticity. The student does not have to worry about the sequence of motor movements necessary to form the letters; he merely has to identify which letter is being requested and select the appropriate letter. The experience of focusing *only* on letters and sounds is especially critical for the student who is dyslexic and dysgraphic.

Setup for activity: Give the student the entire array of alphabet letters from which to make choices, or, to simplify the activity, just present the specific

Figure 10.3—The primary roots of English (Henry 1996)

	Sounds	Syllables	Morphemes
Anglo-Saxon	**Consonants** • single • blends • digraphs **Vowels** • short/long • r-controlled • teams • diphthongs	**6 types:** • closed • open • r-controlled • consonant + *le* • vowel team • vowel-consonant-e	compounds inflections
Romance (Latin)	above plus schwa	basic 6 types complex stress patterns	prefixes suffixes roots plurals
Greek	above plus: • ch • ph • y	basic 6 types	**Combining forms** (scientific vocab.) (*micro + meter*) (*psycho + ology*) **Plurals:** crises

letters being utilized. For students having difficulties, it is best to begin by presenting only the necessary letters and then expand the array of letters as the student becomes more comfortable. Having a larger grouping increases the challenge for making the choice and selecting the desired letter.

Activity 1:   Blending

The teacher creates a word using the letter cards and the student sounds out each letter, blends each sound together, and says the word. If key words are utilized, they can be incorporated if the student is struggling to recall the sound for a letter. Chaining can be added, where a student is asked to change one sound and then read the new pattern.

Teacher: Spell *ham* with the letters.
Student: /h/+/a/ That's /ha/, /m/ that makes /ha/+/m/, **ham**.
Teacher: Good. Now change **ham** to **tam**.

Student takes out **h** and puts in **t**: /t+a+m/ **tam**

Activity 2:   Unblending

The teacher says a word and guides the student to segment

each sound. The student then selects the appropriate letter to represent each sound and spells the word. The concept *unblending* refers to the process of auditorily segmenting the sounds in the word. To expand, the teacher then asks the student what the word would be without one of its letters.

Teacher: *ham*
Student: I hear /h/+/a/+/m/ in *ham*.
Student: (selects letters and spells word) *ham*
Teacher: Good. Take out the **h**. What's the word now?
Student: *am*
Teacher: Is that a real word?
Student: yes
Teacher: Tell me what it means.
Student: It's like I *am* a kid.
Teacher: Now put the **h** back and read the word.
Student: *ham*
Teacher: Take out **m**. What's the word now?
Student: /hăh/
Teacher: Is that a real word?
Student: no

Activity: Chaining

Chaining involves a sequence of sound substitutions and manipulations. Students begin with one pattern and change it multiple times, making only one change each time. Chaining can be performed using letter cards, letter tiles, or small colored blocks to represent the sounds. When using colored blocks, a color does not represent a specific sound, but rather the different colors just represent sameness or difference among sounds. For example, a pattern like *pip* could be represented by three sounds, with the first and last being the same color and *kip* would be represented by three different colors. Chaining patterns can be performed at any level within the sequence, and some examples follow. As in the examples above, it is beneficial to periodically ask the student to determine if a word is a real word, and if so, to define or use the word.

To integrate this type of work with thematic units being used in the classroom, the initial base word can be a word that is relevant to the curriculum. Although integration may be more difficult at this early level when only a few letters are being used, it is fairly easy when working at the higher levels with complex syllables or multi-syllabic words. When selecting words to chain, use the basic sequencing guideline of making only one change each time. Once students understand the concept and the procedures, it is best to vary activities between single-syllable and multi-syllabic patterns.

Chaining at the level of two sound patterns—an example of patterns students are asked to represent:

am	ap	fi
im	ak	ki
it	af	ik
ip	if	ak

Chaining at the CVC level—an example:

tam	*pap	mif
mam	fap	mit
map	fam	tim
tap	maf	dim

*Note: Repetition of a sound necessitates the same color block.

Notice that a change can occur at the initial, final, or middle position, or the sounds can be reversed. Initial changes are usually the easiest for students, followed by final, middle, and reversal changes.

Chaining with CVC-e patterns—two examples:
This cannot be initiated until students are familiar with all of the short vowel sounds and have moved on to long vowel sounds. If appropriate for the students, digraphs or complex syllables containing consonant blends can be added. The long sound is represented by only one symbol or colored block. If using letter cards or tiles, the long sound can be marked as **ā, a-e**, or **ae**. For example, **mate** is only three sounds: /m+ae+t/.

mate	tome
pate	pome
pote	home
vote	hime
*tote	rime

plate	riech
prate	raech
prite	rate
brite	grate
rite	*trate

*Note: Repetition of a sound necessitates the same color block.

Chaining at the complex syllable level, CCVC—an example:

prim	brit	grot
pram	blit	grip
bram	glit	grape
brat	glot	trape

Chaining at the complex syllable level, CVCC—an example:

mast	mist	kapt
past	kist	rapt
pest	kilt	rupt
mest	kipt	ript

A discussion point: Periodically discuss if a word is a real word. When presenting a sound pattern like /kist/ the students may say that it is a real word. Following is a sample dialogue regarding this issue:

Student:	/kist/ is a real word.
Teacher:	What does it mean?
Student:	Like, I *kissed* my mom.
Teacher:	You are right, *kissed* is a real word. When we spell it k-i-s-t then it accurately represents the sounds. But the real spelling of the word is k-i-s-s-e-d.

Chaining at the complex syllable level, CCVCC—an example

skipt	drapt	krift
skapt	draft	krist
srapt	drift	krisp
trapt	prift	krips

Chaining at the complex syllable level, CCCVCC—an example*:

splats	struks	struks
sprats	strukt	truks
strats	skrukt	twuks
struts	strukt	twusk

*Note: If a sound appears twice within a pattern, the same color block is used. Sounds can be omitted.

Chaining with a variety of complex syllables—*two examples:

grape	*strimps
grap	*strips
grapt	*straps
grat	*strasp
prat	*strast
sprat	*trast
sprot	*trest
sprok	*trent
*sproks	*trept
*spros	*tept
*spres	*taept (taped)

*Note: Remember that a repeated sound within a pattern requires a repeated color.

Activity: Word Families

This activity is useful to help students enhance their visual discrimination to distinguish similar letters and to help them identify and recognize patterns among words.

Setup for activity: Give the student a set of word cards containing two similar word families. For example, at the early level of the sequence, when focusing on CVC words, the student may be given a set of 20 word cards, with each word ending in either **-ap** or **-ad**. To increase the complexity, have the words end in **-ap**, **-ad**, or **-ab**.

The student takes these 20 cards, mixed in random order, and separates them into the two or three different word families. Then the student reads the words in each pile. This activity can also be modified by dictating the words to the student and having her spell the words within each family, placing each family in a different column. This spelling can be verbal, in writing, using air writing, or using a keyboard. As an alternative activity, the student can perform a motor activity such as jumping on a small trampa (36" round rebounder or exerciser), walking on a balance beam, or tapping a small suspendable ball while reading words or orally spelling dictated words.

Activity: Syllabification

It is very important for students to understand basic syllabification rules. A mnemonic picture can be used to represent the six most common rules. The mnemonic *Seven puppies in a circle planted numbers in the sunshine* (Figure 10.4) uses an example word to represent each rule. A full-page version of Figure 10.4 is included on page 197.

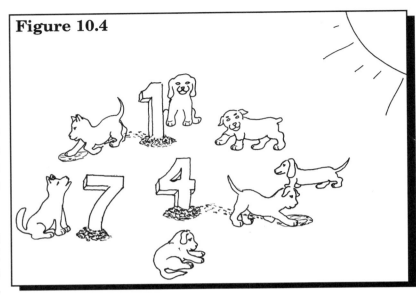

Figure 10.4

Pages 191-192 present the six rules of syllabification plus additional hints. Explanations of these rules can be simplified for younger students and elaborated upon for older students. Older students can include an extra word (paper) to represent both parts of Rule 5. The mnemonic phrase would then be *Seven puppies in a circle planted* paper *numbers in the sunshine*. Additional rules in more elaborated form are available in many multisensory phonics programs. (Gillingham 1968, Henry 1996, Slingerland 1977)

Following is an example dialogue to use in presenting the Syllable Mnemonic:

Teacher:	What do you see here?
Student:	dogs
Teacher:	Right, but these are little dogs.
Student:	oh, puppies
Teacher:	I'll write *puppies* on the board (do so). How many puppies are there?
Student:	seven
Teacher:	Good, I'll write *seven* on the board (do so). What else do you see?
Student:	one
Student:	four
Student:	seven
Teacher:	Good. What are these called?
Student:	numbers
Teacher:	I'll write *numbers* on the board (do so). Can you tell what the puppies did with the numbers?
Student:	digging
Teacher:	Good. But what else?
Student:	making them stand up
Student:	Planting! They're planting the numbers.

Teacher:	Good. What would we say if they already did it?
Student:	planted
Teacher:	Right. I'll put *planted* on the board (do so). What's this in the corner?
Student:	sunshine
Teacher:	Yes. I'll add *sunshine* to our list (do so). Let's see what words we have: *puppies, seven, numbers, planted, sunshine.* Can anyone make a sentence with these words? Start with *Seven puppies.*
Student:	Seven puppies planted numbers in the sunshine.
Teacher:	Good. What else can you add—about how the puppies are? Are they in a line?
Student:	They're in a circle.
Teacher:	Good. Let's add that: *Seven puppies in a circle planted numbers in the sunshine.* (Students repeat.) Now we can use this sentence to help us remember the six ways to divide a word into syllables. (Review *syllable.*) Each word in this sentence will help us remember one rule.
	The first rule is about a compound word. (Review *compound word.*) In a compound word, the word is divided between the two real words. What word in our sentence is an example of this rule?
Student:	sunshine
Teacher:	Good (writing). We can divide it like this: sun/shine. (Continue with the remaining rules.)

Activity 1: **Syllable chaining**

Chaining activities are very useful when used with syllabification. It is important that students become aware of common prefixes and suffixes, and these should be taught as separate activities. Pointing out common prefixes and suffixes in content area words throughout the curriculum is a very useful way to continually reinforce these concepts.

Syllable chaining can be performed in a variety of ways.
- Syllable chaining using colored squares
  Students each have several small squares of colored paper or felt, about three inches square. The teacher states a word and students represent each syllable of the word by using a different colored square for each syllable (represented by the initial of the color in the example).

An example:

Teacher: *sun shine*

Student: (tapping) That's two chunks: 🅡 🅖. (Student says the word and taps each block as that syllable is said.)

Teacher: Change *sunshine* to *Sunday*.

Student: (tapping) That's two chunks and the second one changed: 🅡 🅑. (Student says the word and taps each square as that syllable is said.) *sunshine, Sunday*

Teacher: Change *Sunday* to *funday*.

Student: (tapping) That's two chunks and the first one changed: 🅨 🅑. (Student says the word and taps each square as that syllable is said.)

Teacher: Change *funday* to *fundation*.

Student: (tapping) That's three chunks and you added one to the end: 🅨 🅑 🅡. (Student says the word and taps each block as that syllable is said.) *fundation*

Variation: If accenting has been taught, the student can then determine which syllable is the accented syllable and identify it by raising that square slightly higher than the others.

Variation: Students can analyze the sounds within the stressed (accented) syllable. It is useful to focus only on identifying the sounds in the stressed syllable because these sounds are usually truer and do not degrade to a schwa sound. English has many examples where unstressed syllable sounds are pronounced with slight variations.

Activity 2: **Syllable chaining with letter and syllable cards**
A combination of cards can be used. Some cards contain individual letters and some contain a prefix or suffix. Students can create words using these syllables. Variations include:

- Students create their own words and pronounce them.
- The teacher dictates a word which students create. The teacher dictates alternatives (chaining), changing only one syllable at a time. Example chains follow. Periodically ask students to identify any real words they hear in the patterns.

- After each chaining activity, have students read and write to dictation a few of the words. This is critical to promote integration.

An example of syllable chaining:

res pir a tion	cer tain
res pir a tor	cer tain ly
res pir a tor y	un cer tain
as pir a tor y	un cer tain ly
as pir a tor	*as cer tain
con pir a tor	as cer tain able
con spir a tor	as tain able

*Discuss what happens to the accent and vowel sounds in this change.

Activity 3: **Decoding multi-syllablic words**
It is useful for students to learn a systematic approach when decoding a multi-syllablic word. This strategy should be practiced to the point of automaticity using words in a list, and it should be reviewed and reinforced whenever introducing new vocabulary related to curriculum content. When the student has practiced and developed automatic use of the strategy, then he will be ready to confidently and independently apply the strategy to words he encounters in context.

The strategy consists of three steps:
1) Identify and mark each vowel sound.
   Examples: independence
             approach
             comfortable

Then identify if the vowel is long or short or silent as in **ĭndēpĕndĕncé**.

Students may cross out a silent vowel, as in **comfortablé** or **independencé**.

2) Identify and circle any word ending (suffix).
   Examples: indepen(dence)
             comfor(table)

3) Divide the word into syllables.
   Examples: ap/pr<u>o</u>ach
                 c<u>om</u>/f<u>or</u>t/<u>able</u>

Some students find it easier to work from the right in identifying the syllables.

<u>indepen</u>/dence   <u>inde</u>/pĕn/dence   ĭn/dē/pen/dence

After applying the three steps to a word, the student pronounces the word. He may need to modify or flex some sounds to help himself recognize the word. For example, if the first syllable in *approach* is pronounced with a heavy /p/ sound, the word sounds funny. In flexing the sounds, the student adjusts the sounds (in this case, the /p/ sound) and tries the word again.

Practicing Decoding and Encoding

This section describes sample activities that can be used to help the students practice decoding and encoding in a variety of situations and games throughout the day. The following activities are included merely as suggestions and springboards for ideas a teacher may wish to develop. These activities can be varied or included within a thematic unit revolving around given key words.

Activity1:   Decoding charts
These examples combine blending with a visual tracking strategy, thus enhancing the overall positive effects of the activity.

For these activities, the students use choral reading. The teacher prepares a chart, focusing on a specific sound or blend. To work with groups, a chart having five to ten rows, but only five columns, is useful. Sounds should be selected that are familiar to the students. (Note: In the example below, the columns are numbered only to facilitate explanations.)

1	2	3	4	5
m	n	p	a	t
c	h	t	a	m
l	s	d	a	d

The students read CVC (consonant-vowel-consonant) words containing three sounds. They read from each line three times, changing the initial sound each time. Following is the sequence using the chart on the previous page.

- Read the sound /m/ (column 1). Read the sound /a/ (column 4). Read the sound /t/ (column 5). Blend the sounds: /m/+/a/+/t/ *mat*

- Read the sound /n/ (column 2). Read the vowel sound /a/ (column 4). Read the final consonant /t/ (column 5). Blend the sounds: /n/+/a/+/t/ *(nat)*.

- Read the consonant sound for /p/. Read /a/. Read /t/. Blend the sounds: /p/+/a/+/t/ *(pat)*.

Students then continue reading until they have read through all the lines in this manner. The chart can be varied so that different sounds become the variable sound, as in the full-page, ready-to-use charts on pages 193-195. A key is included on page 196.

Activity 2: **Clapping syllables and other sponges**
Syllable clapping is a good activity to use in the small time units which are found in any classroom, sometimes called *sponge time*. When a teacher has one or two minutes before dismissal, it is useful to pull in a specific reinforcement activity and use this as the structure for dismissal or grouping. Sponges can be performed with an individual or as a group activity. Although it is harder to monitor the specific performance of each individual student when the activity is done within a group, it is not impossible.

Example of using a sponge as structure for dismissal:
- All students whose names start with /m/ may line up.

- Students who have /ă/ in their names may come to the circle.

- Johnny, fist the syllables in the word *establishment*. (He does so.) Good, you may get your lunch.

Examples of other sponges include:
- State a word. Students clap (or fist) the syllables. While doing so, they should focus on feeling the sequence of sounds in their mouths. Note: When fisting the syllables, students tap the table with their fist as they say each syllable.

- State a word. Students state the first sound.
- State a word. Students state the final sound.
- State a word. Students state the medial sound.
- State a word and ask a student to substitute a sound. Example: Say *moose*. Take off /m/ and add /g/. (*goose*)
- Ask students to feel the accenting within a word: "Place your hand under your chin. As you say the word, the accented syllable will cause your chin to come down farther than the others."
- State three or four sounds. Ask students to blend the sounds to discover the word. Example: /s/+/l/+/ee/+/p/ (*sleep*)
- Ask students to think of a two-syllable word that has a double consonant in the middle.

Activity 3: **Charades**

Each student in the group is given a card with an alphabet letter on it. The letters can be chosen to emphasize those the teacher wishes to review. The students form a semi-circle and one student draws a big **a** on the chalkboard and says, "A is for (ant)," naming any example word. The student who has the letter **a** moves to the center and performs a movement to represent a different word beginning with **a**. The student needs to perform the movement through charades or miming, without using any words. The rest of the group attempts to guess her word. For example, "apple" might be communicated by pretending to pick an apple, rub it off, and bite into it. After the students correctly guess the word, both students return to their places in the semi-circle and the activity continues with another letter. Older students might add humor, satire, and puns within their activity.

As an alternative, ask one student to chose a letter of the alphabet, and have the group brainstorm as many nouns (or verbs or adjectives) they can think of that begin with that letter within a period of two minutes. The group then chooses one of the most unique words, and a student is selected to demonstrate the meaning of that word through mime and movement. This can be performed in small groups, with each group miming for another group who tries to guess the word.

Reading Fluency

Students are able to achieve greater and more efficient fluency when reading if they do not have to stop and decode individual words. Three of the ways that can be used to achieve this goal are:

- Previewing the text
- Studying aloud
- Using the TREAT technique

Activity 1: **Previewing the text**

Students can preview the text by scanning each sentence, looking for words that may be difficult. These can be written in a list, analyzed using the three-step strategy, and practiced. When the student feels comfortable, she then reads the whole paragraph or text. Using this technique, the student will be able to read the passage more fluently because she will be familiar with the difficult words. The key is to be sure the student analyzes each word, thereby creating a cognitive link.

When first using this technique, the student should begin with only one or two paragraphs at a time. As she becomes more proficient, she can then progress to larger chunks.

Activity 2: **Studying aloud**

This technique allows the teacher to monitor how well students are applying their decoding knowledge. The students read each story twice; the first time is for **studying** and the second is for **pleasure** and **fluency**.

In a small group, the students take turns reading one or two sentences. The first student reads the first sentence aloud and is told, "Try to phrase the words together by looking ahead a little bit. If it doesn't sound right, you can read it again." The student goes to the next sentence only after he is satisfied with the first.

The students take turns throughout the whole paragraph or passage, with the teacher's assistance in correcting any errors. Then the students, either as a group or taking turns, reread the whole passage or story. The purpose at this point is to read for pleasure, fluency, and comprehension.

Activity 3: **The TREAT technique**

TREAT is an acronym for the *Tactile Reading Eidetic Auditory*

Technique. It combines proven learning strategies to strengthen specific reading skills. Using a multisensory approach, TREAT is a powerful tool to enhance motivation while developing reading fluency, automatic decoding, and comprehension for students who struggle with reading.

Timing and Use: Sessions may vary between 15 and 30 minutes each. For maximum effectiveness, use regularly two or more times weekly. However, TREAT may be helpful even when used only once or twice monthly. This technique can be used with any age student who meets the prerequisites.

Prerequisites:
1. Student is familiar with basic sound/symbol associations.
2. Student can decode words at approximately first grade level.

Guidelines: The TREAT program comprises four sequential steps. It is valuable to closely follow the guidelines for maximum benefit. The steps are as follows:
1. Establish the baseline
2. Tactile and/or visual stimulation
3. Timed reading
4. Repeat reading

Step 1: Baseline
Establish a words-per-minute baseline. This motivates students by letting them see their progress. The student reads material at or slightly below the normal reading level. Record words-per-minute, material used, and an error analysis (substitutions, reversals, omissions, transpositions, and so forth) for future comparison. Take the baseline for four minutes. Determine comprehension by asking questions involving facts, the main idea, and topic analysis. For students with attentional problems, four minutes may be too long. A shorter time interval may be used, as long as that interval is used consistently for both the baseline and the progress testing.

Step 2: Stimulation
Use plastic letters to provide visual and/or tactile stimulation. This increases the student's use of eidetics or visualization skills (automatic visual recall of letter combinations). Cover

one or both eyes and have the student trace, copy, or handle alphabet letters while naming each letter and its primary sound. Do *not* omit this step, even if the letter names and sounds are fully automatic. It does not seem to matter whether the student traces the letter with a finger, copies it, or identifies it by tactile means, so the activity should be varied during alternate practice sessions. The following criteria can help determine which eye and hand to select (Bakker et al 1990), although variation is more important than sticking with only one side:

- Use the right hand and/or the right eye if a student reads below grade level, reads slowly, and/or reads with lack of fluency, jerkiness, or uneven pausing.

- Use the left hand and/or the left eye if the student reads quickly, skips letters or words, and/or reverses letters or words.

Cover both eyes occasionally and have the student use tactile methods to identify the letters. If the dominant hand was not chosen, do not have the student use a pencil to copy. Tracing with the fingers and tactile identification can be done with the non-dominant hand.

Alphabet materials may include sandpaper letters, three-dimensional letters, indented letters such as Ideal's *Groovy Letters*, or plain manuscript letters printed by the instructor. If three-dimensional letters are purchased, accurate shape is important; some commercial letters are poor manuscript representations. Variable methods of stimulation are valuable to provide a variety of tactile and visual integration skills and to encourage generalization.

If the stimulation technique is used more than three times weekly, single-eye occlusion should be intermittent. Covering one eye too frequently for training risks interference with binocular skills and should be used sparingly by educators.

Step 3: Timed Reading (Progress Testing)
After stimulation, the student reads aloud for four minutes. Use new material that is at the same reading level as the baseline material. Record words-per-minute and the error analysis. As the student progresses, establish baselines using higher level materials.

Step 4: Repeat Reading

Perform 5 to 15 minutes of repeat reading. Follow this step *closely*, selecting reading material that is slightly challenging to the student. The instructor reads aloud, pointing to each word while the student follows visually. The instructor may read as little as one word or as much as an entire page at one time, depending on the student's ability to recall the visual and auditory input. The initial reading by the instructor is important. The instructor's model allows the student to experience success by repeating correctly, fluently, and with an awareness of punctuation. If the student has strong auditory memory, some words may be remembered instead of decoded, contributing to fluency. Watching the finger point to each word strengthens eidetic processes.

After the instructor reads as much as a student can repeat with 90 to 100% accuracy, the student rereads the same material aloud. Again the instructor points to each word. The instructor's finger stops only if a word is missed or skipped. In this way, the student receives immediate nonverbal feedback at each error and is cued to reread the word. Continue and complete the reading section.

Repeat reading helps the student maintain a smoother reading pattern, especially if there are tracking or eye movement problems. Give positive feedback frequently; a soft "good" or "great" will not interrupt reading. Repeat the cycles of instructor reading/student rereading.

Syllable Division Rules

❶ Compound words—the word is divided between the two words

sun/shine   play/ground
bed/time   milk/shake
wish/bone   base/ball

❷ Double consonant words—divide between two consonants

pup/pies   kit/ten
hap/py   but/ter
din/ner   ham/mer

❸ Consonant **-le** words—the consonant before **-le** is included in the syllable

cir/cle   can/dle
lit/tle   ap/ple
puz/zle   scuf/fle

❹ Words ending in **-ed** after a final **d** or **t**—the **-ed** forms a syllable

plant/ed   mend/ed
land/ed   hunt/ed
rust/ed   blast/ed

❺ Words with a consonant between two vowels—
   a) When the consonant goes with the second syllable, the first vowel is usually long.

      pa/per   bro/ken
      pu/pil   mu/sic
      spi/der   clo/ver

   b) When the consonant stays with the first syllable, the first vowel is usually short.

      sev/en   cop/y
      trav/el   nev/er
      hab/it   riv/er

Syllable Division Rules

❻ Words with two different consonants between two vowels—
the word is usually divided between the two consonants

num/bers   bas/ket
pen/cil   un/der
sis/ter   af/ter

Other hints:

❶ If a syllable ends in a vowel, the vowel sound is usually long
(open syllable).

ta/ble   ba/by   de/light   e/ven

❷ If a syllable ends in a consonant, the vowel sound is usually
short (closed syllable).

rab/bit   sev/en   in/form   bas/ket

❸ When two vowels are together in a word and both vowels
are heard, divide between the two vowels (divide between
vowels which do not make a single vowel sound).

qui/et   di/a/monds   vi/o/let   zo/o/lo/gy

❹ Do not divide between a digraph (two vowels or two consonants that create a single sound: ea, ai, ck, sh).

buck/les   freck/le   rath/er

❺ Prefixes and suffixes are usually separate syllables.

en/large/ment   de/crease   at/tach/ment

Definitions:

Prefix:	a letter or syllable added to the beginning of a word to modify the meaning of the word
Suffix:	a letter or syllable added to the end of a root word to modify the meaning of the word
Open syllable:	a syllable that ends in a vowel having a long sound
Closed syllable:	a syllable that ends in a consonant and has a short vowel sound

Chart 1: Reviewing a Single Vowel, Initial Sounds Change

m	n	p	a	t
c	h	t	a	m
l	s	d	a	d
s	g	l	a	s
g	t	n	a	b
b	f	r	a	n
s	l	w	a	g
p	r	j	a	m
n	g	r	a	p
b	f	c	a	t

Chart 2: Reviewing Multiple Vowels, Final Sounds Change

d	i	n	p	g
l	e	d	g	n
t	a	p	b	n
t	u	g	m	b
s	i	n	p	t
r	o	b	t	n
m	e	t	n	sh
r	a	m	p	t
d	i	p	m	sh
c	o	t	p	d

The Source for Dyslexia & Dysgraphia
Copyright © 1999 LinguiSystems, Inc.

Chart 3: Reviewing Blends, Final Sounds Change

c	l	a	p	d	n
b	l	o	ck	t	nd
c	r	a	b	ck	sh
f	l	a	t	sh	ck
b	r	i	ck	m	sk
p	r	o	d	m	p
t	r	a	p	mp	m
b	l	a	b	nd	st
d	r	u	m	g	nk
f	l	a	g	t	x

Decoding and Encoding Figures

mat	nat	pat
cam	ham	tam
lad	sad	dad
sas	gas	las
gab	tab	nab
ban	fan	ran
sag	lag	wag
pam	ram	jam
nap	gap	rap
bat	fat	cat

din	dip	dig
led	leg	len
tap	tab	tan
tug	tum	tub
sin	sip	sit
rob	rot	ron
met	men	mesh
ram	rap	rat
dip	dim	dish
cot	cop	cod

clap	clad	clan
block	blot	blond
crab	crack	crash
flat	flash	flack
brick	brim	brisk
prod	prom	prop
trap	tramp	tram
blab	bland	blast
drum	drug	drunk
flag	flat	flax

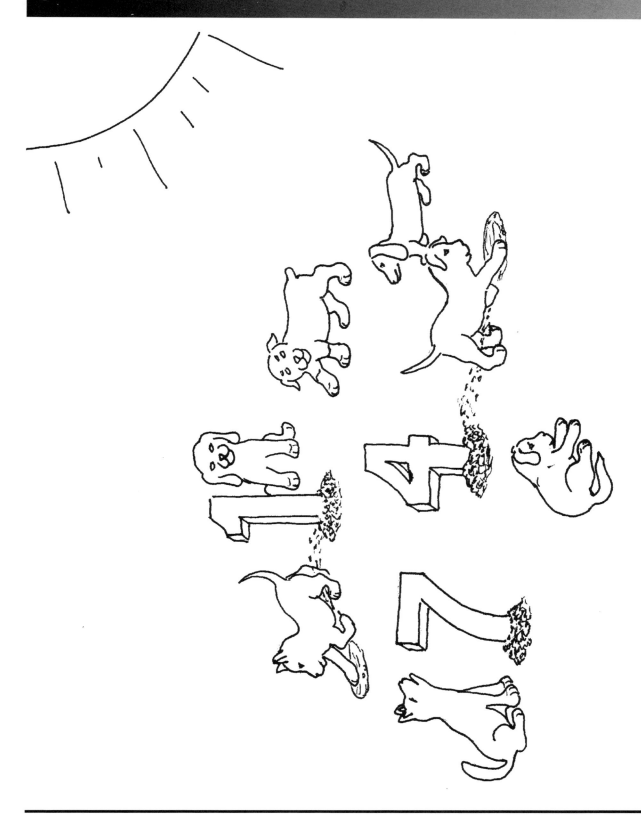

Chapter 11

Spelling

Multiplicity of Spelling Patterns

Since many dyslexics struggle with rote recall, especially rote sequential recall, it helps if they have an **understanding** of the concept behind what needs to be memorized. One of the concepts that is important in spelling is to understand the multiplicity of sound/symbol associations in English. The English language is a phonetic language; we use the alphabetic system wherein sounds are represented by a single letter or letter combination. However, because English has been derived from many other languages, we have a wide variety of visual configurations. Words derived from other languages often retain their visual configuration, such as **ph**, **mn**, and vowel **y**. It is valuable to help students use mnemonics for sounds that can be represented by more than one letter or letter combination as in Chapter 9. In addition, it is useful for students to be helped to develop some basic insights into the spelling process.

The Six Acquired Insights

Spelling development cannot be tightly sequenced because it is very dependent upon each child's reading ability and the specific instructional methods used. (Levine 1998) Rather than calling the steps *sequences to development*, Levine uses the term *acquired insights*. For some children, some of the insights will occur as parallel developments, especially insights number three and four. However, the precise interaction will depend on the child's learning style, reading ability, specific instruction used, and the existence of any learning difficulties (what Levine calls *developmental dysfunctions*) that interrupt the child's use of decision-making clues.

The following presents Levine's six acquired insights along with sample recommendations on how to enhance development at each level.

Insight I: Pre-conventional spelling
What it is:
1. Emerges at about the time preschoolers imitate writing
2. Preschoolers become aware that there is spelling

and they develop a basic awareness that there are sounds and that sounds create words.
- Spellings appear bizarre, but have logic of their own.
  Example: *bgan* for began; *drsr* for dresser
- Spellings include many omissions and substitutions.

How to enhance:
1. Early literacy levels of phonological awareness
   a. Level 1: Rhyming and Alliteration
   b. Level 2: Sound Awareness and Rhyming Production
   c. Level 3: Sequencing Sentences into Words
2. Discovery techniques to kinesthetically feel a sound as it is said, first sounds in isolation and later sounds within a syllable

Insight II: Growing awareness of grapheme-phoneme relationships
What it is:
1. Mastery of the alphabet
2. Sensitivity to a logical system of phonetic equivalency
3. Spellings are more phonetic, e.g., *rite* for write
4. Errors are logical regarding grapheme-phoneme correspondences

How to enhance:
1. More advanced auditory levels of phonological awareness
   a. Level 4: Auditory Blending and Analysis
   b. Level 5: Syllable Segmentation
   c. Level 6: Phoneme Segmentation
   d. Level 7: Phoneme Manipulation
2. Sound/symbol correspondence using mnemonics, such as MFR
3. Use of consistent key words
4. Chaining activities using colored blocks or construction paper
5. Use of invented spelling to monitor development

Insight III: Integration of language
What it is:
1. Greater awareness of morphology and syntax
2. Greater awareness of linguistic cues
   a. Root words
   b. Effects of syntax
   c. Metalinguistic awareness
3. Increased vocabulary understanding and usage

How to enhance:
1. More advanced phonological awareness activities

    a. Level 7: Phoneme Manipulation
    b. Level 8: Syllable Manipulation
2. Syllable chunking or fisting
3. Recognition of morphological markers (units of meaning in words)
4. Blending and unblending patterns and chaining techniques
5. Use of electronic spell checker to hook together (integrate) phonetic analysis and eidetics
6. SAGE technique as on page 204

Insight IV: Application of rules
What it is:
1. Some rules gained by deduction
2. Some rules directly taught
3. Rules integrated with decision making
4. Phonetic analysis integrated with visual eidetics

How to enhance:
1. More advanced phonological awareness activities, including Level 8: Syllable Manipulation
2. Syllable rules
3. Ending rules and recognition of suffixes
4. Spelling rules
5. Multi-syllabic chaining techniques
6. Mnemonic tricks for tricky spelling areas as on page 208

Insight V: Enhanced visualization
What it is:
1. Requires different aspects of memory
    a. Visual recognition memory
    b. Visual sequential memory
    c. Retrieval memory
    d. Spatial memory
2. Good spellers need to recall visual configurations of words of increasing length and complexity.
3. Sight word growth is based on knowledge of rules, regularity, and patterns.
4. Incorporates monitoring skills and attention to detail

How to enhance:
1. More advanced phonological awareness activities, including Level 9: Higher Levels of Phoneme Syllable Manipulation
2. Memory aids for tricky words
3. Imagery and visualization techniques, as in SAGE

4. Multisensory activities
5. Visual activity charts, as in Chapter 10

Insight VI: Automaticity
What it is:
1. Ultimate objective: spell accurately while doing something else, like writing a sentence
2. Student has an increasingly larger storehouse of words available for automatic retrieval.
3. Automaticity is needed to liberate memory, attention, and cognition to engage in more sophisticated intellectual and creative enterprises.

How to enhance:
1. Practice, practice, practice
2. Make sure lower level skills are adequate
3. Compensate for reduced active working memory, if necessary

Many dyslexics and dysgraphics may only achieve to Insight IV or V. They can learn to memorize spelling words for their weekly spelling tests; however, they often do not generalize spelling accuracy into their daily written work. The reason these students struggle to move spelling into automaticity is because of their processing gaps. It is critically important, therefore, to provide the dyslexic student with tools to enhance spelling. These include mnemonics for important, frequently-used words plus a strong system for phonetically logical spelling, thus enabling the student to use electronic aids. With these tools, the dyslexic or dysgraphic student, while never reaching true automaticity, is able to produce a well-spelled paper when the situation demands.

Electronic Spell Checker

The Franklin Company has a line of products they refer to as electronic reference products. These handheld devices accept words spelled phonetically and then display probable matches. An added benefit for dyslexics is a unit with a speaking component to help ensure the words are correctly read, such as the Language Master 6000, which is this author's personal favorite for students. For many, the Franklin Language Master® is more useful than a spell checker on a computer because many spell checkers on a computer match words based on the initial letters, with some exceptions, such as f/ph. For example, both a spell checker on a computer (WordPerfect 6.1®) and the Franklin Speller (Language Master 6000) identified a correct spelling option for the misspellings such as: *fizishin* (physician) and *fotogruf* (photograph). However, misspellings for *knew* (noo) and *food* (fud) were not identified by a computer, although they were identified by the Franklin. Some of the options given by the Franklin Language Master for *noo* and *fud* were as follows:

no	know	no way	new	gnu	knew	noon
nook	(plus 14 more)					

food	feud	fad	fed	fade	feed	fund
fun	fur	fwd	feuds	foods		

Three main aspects contribute to the success of a Franklin Language Master for dyslexic and dysgraphic students, not only as a compensation but also as a remedial technique. These three aspects are analysis, eidetics, and the process of decision making.

Analysis

The analysis aspect is very important. The student thinks of a word, says the word, and then predicts how it is spelled based on logical analysis of the sounds. This helps the student pull in and reinforce what he has learned regarding phonetic analysis: sound/symbol correspondence, prefixes, suffixes, and syllabification. Actually making the prediction helps the student move systematically through the process of problem solving to spell the given word.

Eidetics

Eidetics are an important part of automatic reading and involve easy recognition of letter forms as well as sequences of letters. For example, *-tion* should be an automatic eidetic recognition for the common suffix pronounced /shun/. Eidetics for spelling involve automatic retrieval of common patterns, a process which is hard to develop for dyslexics. By seeing the choices of words given in the Franklin Language Master®, the student develops and reinforces eidetic processing to help future recognition and retrieval of the word. This creates an aspect of visual discovery for the student. The "say" button is valuable to compensate whenever the student is unsure of the pronunciation of a given word, whether in the word list or within the definition.

Decision making

As the student selects the word from the list of choices, he participates in an aspect of decision making which is very valuable in eliminating wrong choices as well as in selecting the correct choice. The process of making the choice helps the dyslexic student develop firmer, more consistent, and more automatic eidetics. This aspect utilizes a higher form of problem solving than mere guessing.

Activity: **SAGE: Spelling Analysis and Generalization of Eidetics**

SAGE is an activity designed to help students utilize the process of spelling analysis and, in doing so, develop and generalize visual eidetics. It is especially valuable in enhancing the third spelling insight. There are five steps to the SAGE procedure.

- Define and discuss
- Write and underline
- Check and rewrite
- Check word parts
- Compare and rewrite

Many benefits are derived from the SAGE technique. Among them are:

- Increase comfort with a technological compensation such as the Franklin Language Master®
- Review learned analytical skills
- Increase phonetic spelling of multi-syllabic words
- Generalize use of analytical skills
- Incorporate the analytical skills within vocabulary and knowledge development

Following is a discussion of the steps for SAGE. To begin, the teacher selects a word and uses it in a sentence that is at or slightly above the student's grade level. The sentence should have good cognitive content. If students are also using visual imagery strategies as in *Visualizing and Verbalizing* techniques (Bell 1991), it is useful to select words and sentences from *Vanilla Vocabulary* (Bell 1993) because of the book's organization and structure. Otherwise, select words and sentences from a favorite literature book or from the core curriculum.

Step 1: Define and Discuss

The teacher states the key word. The students chunk the word into syllables by tapping or fisting each syllable (using their fist to lightly pound the table). Then students read the word, with assistance and feedback from the teacher as necessary. The students then try to interpret its meaning. The teacher guides students through discovery questions, using students' knowledge of prefixes and suffixes and leading them to an appropriate definition. The teacher then states her definition.

Step 2: Write and Underline

The teacher dictates a sentence containing the key word. Each student writes the sentence to dictation and then underlines any word(s) she feels may be misspelled. This step is an important aspect to increase students' self-awareness of eidetics as well as proofreading strategies.

Step 3: Check and Rewrite

Each student proofreads her written sentence and attempts to rewrite underlined words using sound analysis procedures. After writing each word, the student reads it as rewritten, first in chunks (syllables), and then blended together. If the word is still not correct, the student moves to step four for that word before writing the next one. If too many words are underlined, the teacher may select two to four words for emphasis, being certain that the key word is included if it was underlined. Since the selected sentence is at or above grade level, there may initially be many underlined words. The teacher judges how many words to include, based on time permitted and student's level.

Step 4: Check Word Parts

Students recheck rewritten words with specific emphasis on word endings, prefixes, and suffixes. This step should never be omitted because it develops important awareness skills and use of critical structured components. This step is especially important with dyslexics since it is common for these students to omit word endings when reading and writing.

Step 5: Compare and Rewrite

Using the selected rewritten words, the student checks each using a tool such as a Franklin Language Master®. The student writes the correct spelling next to the word as initially written using logical phonetic analysis. Students compare and discuss any differences, with emphasis on comparing the phonetic spelling with the traditional spelling. The process of comparison is a critical step for students' learning, especially because it reinforces the logic of the analysis and the correct eidetics. Students then further discuss the meaning to create and reinforce the link between sound analysis, word parts, and word meaning.

Enhancement Steps for SAGE

1. Students select underlined words, other than the primary word, and after correcting any misspellings, they discuss the meaning and look up definitions of these words.

2. Using the original target word, students write a sentence which describes that word's meaning. The sentence should be substantially different from the original dictated sentence.

3. Students use picture imaging and verbalizing procedures to visualize and discuss the meaning of the vocabulary word. (Bell 1991)

Having students visualize the vocabulary has been helpful in many ways, especially since they may use the same procedures for paragraph and story comprehension. The benefit of visualized vocabulary is in utilizing the brain's natural ability to attach meaning to language through images. Nanci Bell and Phyllis Lindamood state in the prefix to *Vanilla Vocabulary* (Bell 1993), "Ask yourself what works in your brain when you think of a concrete word. Try the word *recital*. What happened in your brain? Try an easier word: *horse*. Try *cat*. Are you noticing that you image or visualize? For *recital*, did you see a girl playing a piano, or a boy playing a violin, or an adult playing the cello?" It is possible to see and hear a word and perceive the sounds within a word, but "without an image for meaning, the oral and written symbol is meaningless." Even as a student deals with more abstract words, the meaning is still, in some aspect, imaged. For example, for the meaning of *freedom*, we can image animals free in the countryside. We can also use other senses of imagery besides visual imagery. We may imagine a sound, a sensation, or an emotion. Bell and Lindamood state, "The richer and stronger our images, the more solid our grasp of meaning." The use of images helps develop vocabulary, especially in children who learn differently, and who may be very strong in how they process visual, spatial and kinesthetic information to image meaning, activities, and events.

Activity: **Example of a SAGE Activity**
The word *develop* was selected from *Vanilla Vocabulary*, using the definition "to bring, or to come gradually into being." The

sentence used was the first example: "It took several days for the naked baby birds to develop feathers."

Step 1: Define and Discuss
Students are presented with the word *develop*. They chunk it: *de-vel-op* and then read the word. Next, they guess its meaning. Through structured questions, they are guided toward a definition. The teacher then tells them the book's definition.

Step 2: Write and Underline
The teacher dictates the sentence for the students to write. Each student then underlines any words he feels may be misspelled, as in the following example. "It <u>tuk</u> <u>sevrul</u> days for the <u>nakid</u> baby <u>birdz</u> to <u>devlup</u> <u>fethers</u>."

Step 3: Check and Rewrite
Students check each underlined word, rewriting it using analytical skills. For example, *devlup* would be written in syllables, perhaps as *de vel up*.

Step 4: Check Word Parts
For example, in looking at the word "birdz," the student may remember that plural **s** sometimes has the /z/ sound, but is spelled with the letter **s**. The student may refer to a checklist or chart to review word endings. The student then rewrites the word as *birds*.

Step 5: Compare and Rewrite
The student types the word *develup* into the Franklin. The Franklin provides many options, the first of which is the correct spelling *develop*. The student follows the same process for each word.

Visualization
The many different ways of representing one sound can be confusing. The long *i* sound, for example, is represented in all of the following words but in a different way in each: *silo, sight, psychology, cyclone*, and *cider*. On the other hand, a single combination of letters (*ough*) can be pronounced very differently, as in the following words: *cough, furlough, ought, plough*, and *thorough*. The inconsistencies in English might lead one to spell *fish* as "ghoti" if we used the *gh* in "enough," the *o* in women," and the *ti* in "notion."

Students need to understand basic sound and symbol correspondence and realize that there are irregularities within the English system. Students also need to be able to remember a given sequence of letters as related to specific sounds. Good spellers use visualization to an extensive degree; they can "see the letters" in their mind's eyes. There are ways to help students visually remember correctly spelled words, as in the following four steps:

Step 1: Students trace over (accurately and with fluency) a word on a chalkboard repeatedly, using very large letters. They say the name of each letter as they trace it. This exercise provides multisensory input; the students see the shape, say the name, hear the name, and feel the shape while moving over the letters.

Step 2: Students trace the word without touching the chalk to the board, while naming the letters.

Step 3: Students trace the letters in the air, saying the letters as they trace, emphasizing accurate movements.(Refer to Figure 9.3 on page 164.)

Step 4: Students repeat the tracing with their eyes closed.

These or similar steps can be found in many multisensory programs such as Gillingham's *Remedial Training*, Slingerland's *Multisensory Techniques*, and Bell's *Seeing Stars*. After a student finishes step four, ask, "Can you 'see' the word in your mind while you trace the letters in the air?" If the student says yes, he is beginning to visualize and to recall visually. If not, he needs more reinforcement, practice, and encouragement to see the words in his mind's eye. Students' visualization can be enhanced by asking them to pretend that colored Silly String® or colored spaghetti is coming out of their fingertips as they write in the air. Ask questions such as the following:

- Can you see the shadow left by each letter?
- Can you see all the letters?
- Can you see the colors? What color is your letter? Change it to (blue).
- Can you see which letters are tall? Which are they?
- Can you see which letters are short? Which are they?
- Can you see the first letter?
- Can you see the last letter?

Mnemonics

A common classroom activity is for students to memorize spelling words. To help with the words that are trickiest in any given list, students can develop and use mnemonics, which are memory aids to help with recall. The caution with mnemonics is that too many used at a given time can create an overload and can actually end up creating more confusion. Therefore, it is important to select only two or three words, perhaps the most cumbersome, and create mnemonics for those. Each student can select their own troublesome words based on their individual differences.

Caution:	Restrict the number of mnemonics used at any one time.

Students will learn best when they create their own mnemonics. However, many need substantial modeling and practice before they can comfortably create their own patterns. Five basic strategies can be used in developing mnemonics for spelling patterns. Some words can be used with any of several strategies, whereas mnemonics for others may only be easily developed using a given strategy. When presenting this system, initially use only one or two strategies and work with these until students are comfortable with the system. Add more strategies as students become proficient.

Strategy 1: Mispronounce the word to help focus on the individual components.

Emphasize to students that this is not the actual pronunciation of the word, but only a memory trick to help remember the sequence of letters.

Wed-nes-day   ven-ge-ance
to-get-her   extra-or-dinary

Strategy 2: Create a sentence using a related word that contains the same sequence of letters as the target word.

hear: You *hear* with your *ear*.
beach: A *beach* is by the *sea*.
beech: A *beech tree* is in my yard.
calculator: Use a *calculator or* use your fingers.
ninety: *Nine ty*pewriters typed *ninety* times.
minimum: We bought the *mini*car for the *minimum* cost.
tee: *See* the golf *tee*.
tea: I like to *eat* with my *tea*.

Strategy 3: Create a sentence to focus on a specific aspect of the target word. (This strategy differs from strategy #2 because there is no specific related word using the same letter sequences.)

skiing: Use both i's (eyes) in *skiing*.
accustomed: *A* pair of *cc's* chased *us* to *Tom* and *Ed*.
ecstasy: There is no *x* in *ecstasy*.

prophecy: There is no *f* in *prophecy*.
pressed: There is no *t* in *pressed*.
eight: There is no *a* in *eight*.

Strategy 4: Use the word as an acronym and create a sentence where the first letter of each word spells out the target word.

arithmetic: A rat in the house might eat the ice cream.
geography: George Eaton's old grandmother rides a purple horse. Yippee!
bazaar: Balls always zoom across a room.

Strategy 5: Create a sentence that relates the target word to another word based on its root.

muscular: Large *muscles* make you very *muscular*.
intoxication: *Intoxication* is a very *toxic* condition.
scholastics: *Scholastics* are for *scholars* in school.

Reinforcing Spelling

Following is a wide variety of activities that can be incorporated throughout the curriculum to review spelling words and/or spelling of content vocabulary words. Each activity can be performed with a variety of options:

- Each day, the entire class performs one or two activities, with the same activities being practiced each day.

- The class performs one activity every day, Monday through Thursday, using a different activity each day.

- Activities are performed individually, in small groups, or with the whole class.

- Students may be given a choice of activities and choose their preferred activity.

Following is a sample list of activities. Different activities rely on different modalities to enable a teacher to provide variety throughout the week.

- **Create a story.** Use all of the spelling words.
  - ✔ Tell the story to another person, stopping to spell each spelling word.
  - ✔ Create the story as a group project.
  - ✔ Write the story with a blank for each spelling word, and students switch stories, having another student fill in the blanks. Caution: some dysgraphic students may experience great difficulty with this task and will need modifications.

- **Echo spelling.** One student writes the word on the board, using variation in intonation. The class repeats the word, mimicking the same intonation and writes the word on paper.

- **Tape recorder.** The teacher or a student dictates the spelling words, while each student in the group quietly spells the word into a tape recorder. After the entire list is dictated, each student listens to his own taped version, correcting any spelling errors by comparing his taped spelling with the original written list.

- **Categorize words.** Have students determine criteria for categories and categorize the words. Sample categories include:
  - ✔ All words containing eight letters
  - ✔ Words containing more than one **e**
  - ✔ Words containing all short vowels (or all long vowels or a mix of long and short vowels)
  - ✔ Words which are nouns (or verbs or adjectives)

- **Number code.** The teacher or student creates a number code in which all letters of the alphabet are assigned a number. Each student playing the game has a copy of this code.
  - ✔ Students are given a sheet of paper on which all words have been translated into numbers. They use the code to form the spelling words.
  - ✔ Students are given a list of each spelling word, and they transform the words into the number code.

- **Morse code.** Working with a partner, one student taps out one of the spelling words using morse code, and the partner attempts to guess the word.

- **Type words on a computer.**

- **Write words using a variety of colors.**
  - ✔ Write the words using different colors for letters or parts of words that are confusing.
  - ✔ Write the words in large letters and then trace them multiple times, creating a rainbow by using a different color chalk or crayon for each tracing.
  - ✔ Paint the word large using tempura paints and decorate the letters of the word.

- **Visualize.** Close eyes and picture the word on the "chalkboard in your mind" as the teacher or a partner dictates the words.
  - ✔ This can be incorporated with motor activities such as a trampa (36" round rebounder or exerciser) or a balance beam, or with air writing activities.

- **Slow and fast.** The words are written in a list on the chalkboard. The first word is chanted by the class in an extremely slow tempo, with a long delay between each letter. The next word is chanted at a brisk, quick pace. Students read through the rest of the list, alternating fast and slow reading. The teacher should set the pace for each word by directing the class as a conductor.

- **Soft and loud.** The list of spelling words is placed on the board, and the class spells each word orally in unison, varying between soft and loud, as listed below. This activity helps focus on vowels, which are a critical component of any syllable.
  ✔ Vowels are soft, consonants loud.
  ✔ Consonants are soft, vowels are loud.

- **Songs, raps, and chants.**
  ✔ Students take turns making up a sing-song rendition of the spellings of several spelling words.
  ✔ Students work in a group to create a rap to spell the words.
  ✔ Students orally chant the spelling of each word in rhythm to a metronome. The metronome can be set at 48 m, 60 m, or 90 m.
  ✔ Students create a song using as many long ā words as possible. Vary with other sounds.

- **Common songs.** Students can spell their words to the rhythm of a common song, saying the letters instead of the words of the song. Examples are as follows:
  ✔ Three-letter words: *Jingle Bells*
  Examples using *mat* and *rub*:

m	**a**	**t**	**m**	**a**	**t**
Jin-	gle	bells,	jin-	gle	bells

  Jingle all the way

r	**u**	**b**	**r**	**u**	**b**
Oh	what	fun	it	is to	ride

  In a one-horse open sleigh.

  Students actually sing "m-a-t, m-a-t, jingle all the way. r-u-b, r-u-b, in a one-horse open sleigh."

  ✔ Five-letter words: *Row, Row, Row Your Boat*
  ✔ Seven-letter words: *Twinkle, Twinkle Little Star*
  ✔ Seven-letter words: *Michael, Row Your Boat Ashore*

Students write each word three times while listening to classical music. Students are encouraged to tap their feet or tap a rhythm with their non-dominant hand while writing.

- **Large muscle activities.**
  - ✔ Students make up a dance, using a conga line, the stroll, or bunny hop, and they chant the letters to their spelling words while dancing.
  - ✔ Stomp or thrust. Words are written in a list on the chalkboard. Students read the letters of each spelling word in unison and stomp, clap, or thrust an arm or leg according to specific criteria.

    Stomp on each consonant (or vowel).

    Thrust the arm forward on each vowel (or consonant).

    Kick a leg forward on each consonant (or vowel).
  - ✔ Vowel hop. The class reads the letters of each word in unison. When a vowel appears, they make a small hop in place while saying the letter.

    Variation: instead of hopping, the class can be seated and stand up (and sit back down) each time a vowel is said.

    Variation: they can stand up (and sit back down) each time a consonant is said.

    Variation: they begin standing and briefly sit each time a vowel is said.
  - ✔ Students create a body alphabet of letters and pantomime each letter of each spelling word.
  - ✔ Students pantomime the meaning of each spelling word and classmates try to guess at the meaning.
  - ✔ Students take turns reading the letters of the word from a chalkboard or large chart while performing a motor activity.

    Use a trampa (36" round rebounder or exerciser).

    Use a balance beam.

    Hit a suspendable ball.

    Bounce a basketball.

- **Textures.** Students write spelling words on textures or using textures, using their finger instead of a pencil. It is important that they say each letter name as they write it. Use textures such as:
  - ✔ Carpet
  - ✔ Light sandpaper
  - ✔ Chocolate pudding
  - ✔ Whipped cream

- **Self-directed goals.** Students create their own goals for how they will study and learn their spelling words.

- **Independent work.** Students work independently to study the words by selecting two different activities which draw upon different learning preferences.

Metacognitive Break

It is valuable for a teacher to periodically stop and analyze the strategies used in various activities, thus enhancing metacognitive awareness. This sample analysis uses the concept of developing mnemonics. On one side of the chart, strategies beneficial for dyslexics are delineated. On the second side, write a brief description of how the spelling mnemonic activity fits into or utilizes each strategy. When you are done, look at the complete chart on page 215 to compare ideas.

Relevant Strategy	How Strategy is Used in Activity
Multisensory presentations • connects kinesthetic feelings with auditory and visual information • provides interactive involvement	
Connections (connective learning) • connects new information to previous knowledge • builds on what students know	
Metacognitive awareness • understanding of the value of using strategies involves awareness of strategies and use of pre-planning	
Mnemonic strategies • uses memory tricks • creates organization • provides a framework for retrieval	
Imagery • obtaining and retaining a visual image of a letter pattern or an auditory image of a sound pattern	
Rhythm • provides another recall pathway • provides dynamic learning • provides a framework for retrieval	
Positive • achieving feeling of success and being aware of the success	

Mnemonic Activity Chart

Relevant Strategy	How Strategy is Used in Activity
Multisensory presentations • connects kinesthetic feelings with auditory and visual information • provides interactive involvement	Students combine visual patterns with letter sequences and sound patterns, while they focus on feeling the sounds in their mouths: a fri**end** to the **end**.
Connections (connective learning) • connects new information to previous knowledge • builds on what students know	Students connect a new word (**beech**) to a known word (**tree**).
Metacognitive awareness • understanding of the value of using strategies involves awareness of strategies and use of pre-planning	Students work to understand how each of the five spelling mnemonic strategies work so that they are then able to decide which works best with a given word: **Wednesday** works well with a mispronunciation, as **Wed-nes-day**.
Mnemonic strategies • uses memory tricks • creates organization • provides a framework for retrieval	Students use a variety of memory aids to strengthen their recall of words and in the process analyze the words more completely to decide which strategy to use.
Imagery • obtaining and retaining a visual image of a letter pattern or an auditory image of a sound pattern	Visualization is involved for acronyms and in comparing word similarities; in strategy #4, students hold the first letter of each word in mind and visualize it to create the acronym.
Rhythm • provides another recall pathway • provides dynamic learning • provides a framework for retrieval	Students chant or mispronounce words, achieving a rhythmic pattern which provides another hook for recall.
Positive • achieving feeling of success and being aware of the success	Students break activity into smaller increments for greater success, and use of strategies generates more hooks and greater recall.

Chapter 12
The Writing Process: Remedial and Bypass Strategies

When students must focus on writing mechanics while completing a task, they learn less.

Even though students who struggle with writing may spend more time on the assignment than their peers, they understand less because so much of their cognitive attention is diverted to the mechanical processes. The unfortunate consequence is that their belief in their own ability to learn diminishes and eventually they may feel *dumb* or as though they are unable to learn. As they mature, more and more emphasis is placed on expressing knowledge through the written form and the discrepancy between their performances and that of their peers widens.

There are four basic steps to follow when writing is a particular problem for students:

1. Understand the process of writing and what is involved within each level of the process.

2. Determine if writing problems are interfering with learning instead of helping, and identify where the process of writing breaks down for an individual child.

3. Help the student build up skills in a sequential, developmental manner so that each level builds on the successes of the previous levels.

4. Help the student move the process of writing from a level of mechanical drudgery into a level of automaticity that generates excitement, fun, and meaning.

It is important to be aware that there are different types of strategies to help students achieve steps 3 and 4: *remedial* and *bypass* strategies.

Remedial strategies . . .
help a student improve functioning in one or more areas through use of systematic techniques.

Bypass strategies . . .
help a student deal with the problem(s) that interfere with writing by going around the problem through use

of different techniques or technology, or by providing compensations which alleviate the strain and increase the ease of writing.

Remedial Strategies

Remedial assistance can focus on any of a variety of areas. Since the student may have difficulty at any level or levels, it is important for the teacher to analyze where the breakdown is occurring.

Remediation is important because students with learning disabilities do not automatically grasp or automatize many aspects of writing mechanics. They need direct systematic instruction so they can use writing mechanics more efficiently, just as good writers do. For many students, especially dyslexic and/or dysgraphic students, the mechanics are not learned through implicit instruction.

Pre-writing (readiness) activities

Readiness activities can be directly taught as a specific lesson and then can be utilized as warm-ups and writing breaks before and during writing tasks. Students who find writing stressful may benefit from one or more 10-second breaks during a writing activity. Activities similar to these warm-ups are often suggested by occupational therapists to help relieve the stress and relax students' writing hand, frequently with beneficial results on their overall posture.

Brief activities which are best adapted as warm-ups or writing breaks. Typical time for each: 10 seconds

- Shake hands fast but not violently.
- Rub hands together and focus on the feeling of warmth.
- Rub hands on the carpet in circles (or on clothing, perhaps on thighs).
- Fold hands together, interlacing fingers with right thumb over left. Move hands apart a few inches and clasp together again five times. Repeat the process with left thumb over right.
- Use dominant hand to push cap of a ballpoint pen while holding it in that hand.
- Use thumb of dominant hand and click top of a ballpoint pen while holding it in that hand. Repeat using index finger.
- Grip a pencil or pen with thumb and first two fingers in a tripod finger grip. "Walk" the fingers up and down the pencil.

Other warm-up activities. Typical time for each is variable, depending on students.

- Students stand next to their desks with hands palm down on their desks. Keeping their arms straight and palms down, students support their weight on their hands for 5-10 seconds and then rock back and forth to the count of 10.
- Students do "sitting push-ups" by placing each palm on their chair with fingers facing forward. They push down on their hands, lifting the body slightly off the chair.
- Each student keeps his arm and wrist on the desk and *writes* the alphabet using his index finger. Then students close their eyes and repeat.
- Students perform simple finger plays. For example, draw faces on child's fingertips and touch thumb to each finger. Young students can pretend the thumbs are mommy and daddy who are kissing each of their "children" (the other fingers).
- Students roll small balls of clay between their thumb and index finger. Right-handers rotate it clockwise; left-handers counterclockwise.
- Students push toothpicks through the lid of an old margarine tub. (Use of an upside-down paper cup can simplify the task if necessary.) Create shapes on the lid to add variety.

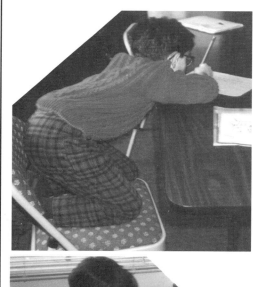

Figure 12.1—Comparison of inefficient and efficient writing postures

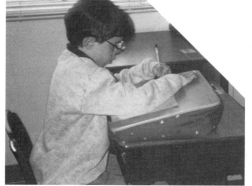

Pencil grip and paper slant

An appropriate pencil grip is critical to enhance writing comfort and ease. It also contributes to increased fluency and automaticity. It would be ideal if all young students could begin their writing experiences with appropriate instruction in these areas. However, if a student has developed inefficient habits regarding grip, it is possible to encourage changes with the appropriate instruction, monitoring, kind reminders, and use of devices such as one of the many plastic or molded pencil grips on the market. However, sometimes for older students, it is more disruptive to try to change ingrained writing habits. If this is the situation, and the inefficient habits interfere with the writing proces, compensations and bypass strategies will be essential.

It is also important to consider the child's overall posture. His feet should rest on the floor (or a box if necessary) rather than hang in the air. The child's arm should rest comfortably on his desk so that he can use fluent movements, as in Figure 12.1 on page 219.

Letter Form: Manuscript

Dysgraphic students benefit by developing fluency in letter form. Some recommendations that can help include air writing and chalkboard practice. This practice is vital for beginning instruction but also very useful as a remedial tool.

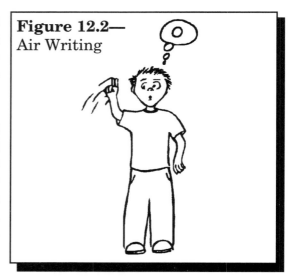

Figure 12.2—
Air Writing

Air writing is most efficient if the student creates large letters in the air, utilizing firm strokes, with elbow and wrist fairly straight. For many students, use of the first two fingers as the pointer or *tip* of the imaginary pencil is very efficient. They pretend that their whole arm is the actual pencil and form large-sized letters. Simultaneous use of verbalizations enhances multi-sensory connections, making them more automatic.

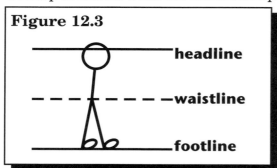

Figure 12.3

headline

waistline

footline

To help students with the relationship of letters, use terms such as *tall letters, waist letters,* and *tail letters* (*headline, waistline* [midline], and *footline*), along with visual and kinesthetic cues that describe the appropriate direction, as in Figure 12.3. For example, an *a* can be a waistline letter (made large with the base at the child's waist), with the verbalization, "Circle around to start, then straight down," or simply, "Around and down." The letter *l* starts at the waistline and goes up to the headline. As the letter form becomes more automatic, the student may say the name and sound as the letter is formed.

Following are some verbal cues that can be used when teaching the letter form. They have been simplified to use a minimum amount of verbiage and, hence, are appropriate for language learning disabled students, including dyslexics.

Manuscript Verbal Cues

a   around and down

b   tall stick down, halfway up, around

c   halfway around

d   around, all the way up, all the way down

e   across, up and halfway around

f   hook to straight line-across

g   around, way down, hook to left

h   tall stick down, halfway up, long hook

i   short stick down-dot

j   line way down, hook to left-dot

k   tall stick down, diagonal in, diagonal out

l   tall stick down

m   short stick down, back up, long hook, back up, long hook

n   short stick down, back up, long hook

o   around in front of your body (RH); around away from your body (LH)

p   way down, back up, half circle to right

q   around in front of your body (RH), way down, hook to right (Note: Teacher can explain, "He wears a tail—he's crazy.")

r   short stick down, back up, hook

s   half circle right, half circle left

t   tall stick down, across

u   short stick down, curve up, back down

v   diagonal down, diagonal up

w   diagonal down, diagonal up, diagonal down, diagonal up

x   diagonal to right (pick up pencil), cross diagonal left

y   diagonal down to right (pick up pencil), diagonal way down left

z   straight line right, diagonal to left, straight line right

As the students air write, encourage them to visualize the letter they have just written. They can pretend they see the *shadow* left by their fingers, that colored spaghetti comes from the end of their fingers, or that their fingers are squirting colored Silly String®. Sometimes have the students close their eyes and air write the letter to determine the efficiency of their motor planning without visual cues.

To enhance the multisensory impact of the air writing activity, have them say the name of each letter as they write it. Chalkboard practice is very valuable for students because it provides practice on a vertical plane. When writing a letter vertically, the direction "up" is always *up* rather than *away from* as it is when writing on a desk.

Guidelines for chalkboard writing are as follows:
- Use large, correctly formed letters, writing at the child's eye level.
- The child traces the letter several times. Using different colors of chalk and calling it *rainbow writing* makes the repetition more fun.
- The child copies the letter several times until the form is correct, using verbal cues as necessary.
- Erase the child's letters, cover up the model, and have the child write the letter without looking at the model.
- Compare the child's letter form to the model.

Letter Form: Cursive Writing
Cursive writing, when performed fluently and with ease, generally reinforces the pattern of syllables and whole words and is often a much quicker writing process. While many students actually perform better using manuscript, many who do could be more efficient using cursive *if* they were taught to do so using a systematic multisensory approach.

Cursive letter form needs to be taught very systematically for dyslexic and dysgraphic students, reinforcing each form with substantial air writing and large chalkboard tracing and copying. Frequent use of reinforcement with rainbow writing is especially beneficial.

Getting Started
1. Evaluate the student's current knowledge of cursive to determine what lowercase letters are known and which are made using correct form (pretest). Unknown or incorrectly made letter forms need to receive the most instruction and emphasis.

2. Teach prerequisite terms demonstrating their meaning using a variety of multisensory techniques (refer to Figure 12.3 on page 220):
   - Cursive
   - Lowercase

- Footline
- Waistline (where you wear your belt—sometimes called midline)
- Headline

The Basic Steps in Sequence

Following are the six steps to follow when teaching the pre-cursive forms or the actual cursive letters. Be sure to review all known letters frequently (ideally daily, if possible).

1. Introduce the form or letter using air writing.
    - The teacher either faces the student (air writing backwards) so the teacher's finger is *leading* each student's finger, or
      The teacher stands behind the student and makes the letter directly next to student.
    - Students use two fingers to point and keep their arms fairly taut.

2. The teacher writes the form or letter large (about 12") on a chalkboard or whiteboard.
    - Students trace the form/letter using the tips of the pointer and middle fingers.
    - Students trace the form/letter using chalk/marker.
    - Students copy the form/letter while looking at the model.
    - Students reproduce the form/letter without a model.

3. Students write the form/letter on large paper copying from a model.
    - If any student's form is not fluent and correct, provide more practice on step 2.

4. Students write the form/letter on large paper without a model.

5. Students write the form/letter on regular-sized primary lined paper.

6. During steps 1-5:
    - Each student says the letter name while tracing or writing.
    - Each student focuses on fluency and correct form.

Pre-cursive Teaching

1. These six basic forms create the basis for all 26 cursive lowercase letters.

2. **Rule**: All single lowercase cursive letters start at the footline.

3. Teach each of the six pre-cursive forms, one at a time. Do not progress to the next form until the child is able to make the form fluently and correctly. Figure 12.4 on page 224 presents all of the forms and corresponding letters.

4. Teach the six forms in this order, using the accompanying label.
   - Tall loop ℓ
   - Short loop e
   - Tall slider ℓ
   - Short slider ι
   - Across the bridge c
   - Up the hill, down the hill n

Figure 12.4

Pre-cursive level	Pre-Cursive Form	Letters
1. Tall loop	ℓ	$\ell\ b\ f\ h\ k$
2. Short loop	e	e
3. Tall slider	ℓ	t
4. Short slider	ι	$i\ j\ p\ r\ s\ u\ w$
5. Across the bridge	c	$c\ a\ d\ g\ o\ q$
6. Up the hill, down the hill	n	$m\ n\ v\ x\ y\ z$

5. Teaching steps for each of the six forms
   - The teacher writes a sequence of three tall loops on board, approximately eight inches high, connected properly to each other.
   - The student uses air writing to trace the tall loops (in air), with the teacher assisting in the motor movements, if necessary. The student may say "loop" or "tall loop" as he air writes.
   - The student traces the tall loop pattern several times, tracing directly over the teacher's model.
   - The student copies the tall loop pattern directly next to the teacher's model.
   - The student practices air writing again.
   - The student writes the tall loop pattern without using a model.

Each student should achieve some degree of automaticity and fluency at each step before progressing to the next. When efficient with a sequence of three forms, the student should repeat the steps using a sequence of six to eight connected forms. Use of a chalkboard is preferable to a whiteboard because there is auditory feedback (from the sound of the chalk moving) along with the visual and kinesthetic feedback provided.

The Cursive Letters

1. The teacher should make sure all letters are properly formed, without extra loops or curls.

2. Teach cursive letters one at a time in the specified sequence. If a student has demonstrated that he already makes one or more letters using the correct form (pretest), then consider those letters as *known*. There is no need to re-teach these letters, but they should be used in reviews.

3. After each letter, teach and practice connections. Have students practice connecting the new letter to each previously taught letter. Demonstrate how a letter loses its ability to start at the footline when it follows a letter with a handle, such as **b**, **o**, **v**, and **w**. Figure 12.5 provides some examples.

Figure 12.5

ba   os   vi   we

4. The sequence for teaching the letters follows the sequence of the six pre-cursive forms:

   - Tall loop   *ℓ*
   - Short loop   *e*
   - Tall slider   *t*
   - Short slider   *i*
   - Across the bridge   *c*
   - Up the hill, down the hill   *m*

- Tall loop   *b*
- Short slider   *j*
- Across the bridge   *a*
- Up the hill, down the hill   *n*

- Tall loop   *f*
- Short slider   *p*
- Across the bridge   *d*
- Up the hill, down the hill   *v*

- Tall loop   *h*
- Short slider   *r*
- Across the bridge   *g*
- Up the hill, down the hill   *x*

- Tall loop   *k*
- Short slider   *s*
- Across the bridge   *o*
- Up the hill, down the hill   *y*

- Short slider   *u*
- Across the bridge   *q*
- Up the hill, down the hill   *z*
- Short slider   *w*

5. Always remember to provide encouragement and positive reinforcement to the students. Focus on what they did *correctly* while gently suggesting any necessary change or adjustment.

Other Mechanical Aspects

It is critical to also teach the other mechanical aspects as separate and distinct steps. Detailed descriptions will not be given here, as there are many efficient programs on the market. The caution is to include specific learning and practice activities; do not assume implicit learning. Areas of focus should include:

- Spacing—between words, after a period, at beginning of a paragraph
- Punctuation
- Capitalization
- Subject/verb agreement
- Parallel grammatical construction (for older students)

Bypass strategies

The overall goal of bypass strategies is to increase automatization and still allow the student to participate in and benefit from the task. If a student can easily manipulate the mechanics, he is free to focus on content. Automatization enhances active working memory, enabling the learner to return to another, perhaps earlier, step in a task and process and integrate it with other elements. This creates ample opportunity for students to focus more completely on the process of writing.

With bypass strategies, the product may be altered, but the student still performs the basic task. The goal is to build in the bypass without negating the idea that handwriting is still important. Valuable bypass strategies which allow the student to go around the problem include:

- **Understanding**—Understand the student's inconsistencies and performance variabilities.
- **Print or cursive**—Allow the student to use either form. Many dysgraphic students are more comfortable with manuscript printing.
- **Computer**—Encourage students to become comfortable using a word processor on a computer. Students can be taught as early as first grade to type sentences directly on the keyboard. In doing so, do not eliminate handwriting for the child; handwriting is still important, but computer skills will be invaluable for longer and important tasks.
- For older students, encourage use of a **speech recognition** program combined with the word processor.
- Encourage consistent **use of a spell checker** on the computer to decrease the overall demands of the writing task.
- Encourage **use of an electronic resource** such as the spell check

component in a Franklin Language Master® to decrease the overall demands. If the student has concurrent reading problems, a Language Master® with a speaking component is most helpful because it will read/say the words.

- Do not count off for poor **spelling** on first drafts, in-class assignments, or on tests.

- If necessary, **shorten** writing assignments.

- Provide the student with a copy of completed **notes** (perhaps through a note-taking buddy who can use carbon paper) to fill in missing parts of her own notes.

- **Staging**—Have students complete tasks in logical steps or increments instead of all at once. This helps decrease demands on active working memory.

- **Prioritization**—Stress or de-emphasize certain task components during a complex activity. For example, students can focus on using descriptive words in one assignment and in another, focus on using compound sentences.

- Allow the student to **tape record assignments** and/or take oral tests.

- Reinforce the **positive aspects** of the student's efforts.

- Be **patient**.

- **Encourage the student to be patient** with himself.

Dysgraphia does not have to limit creativity, as indicated by the sample below, composed on a computer by a 12-year-old dyslexic and dysgraphic student.

a) First draft of creative story as typed by 12-year-old student:
"the way I describe a bumby ride is like wothgan mowtsarts mowsek. eshe bumby rowd is like a song. Eshe bumb is the a note eche uncon at the sam time ste is. that was the mewstere to mowts mowsuk it was vare metereus and unperdekdable.So the next time you drive down a bumby theak of mowtsart."

b) Same story. Student read to teacher using his draft:
"The way I describe a bumpy ride is like Wolfgang Mozart's music. Each bumpy road is like a song. Each bump in the road is a note. Each bump is uncontrolled at the same time it still is controlled. That was the magic to Mozart's music. It was very mysterious and unpredictable. So the next time you drive down a bumpy road think of Mozart."

Compensatory Strategies

The overall goal of compensations is similar to bypass strategies: increase automatization so the student can use the writing process more efficiently. Thus, without changing the content or the product, the compensation can reduce any negative impact that writing has on the child's learning or ability to express knowledge.

Valuable strategies include:

- **Understanding**—Understand the student's inconsistencies and performance variabilities.

- **Print or cursive**—Allow the student to use whichever form is more comfortable.

- Have the student **proofread papers after a delay,** using a checklist of the points to check. If students proofread immediately after writing, they may *read* what they intended rather than what was actually written.

- If getting started is a problem, **encourage pre-organization strategies**, such as use of graphic organizers.

- Allow **extra time** for writing activities.

- **Note taking**—Provide a partially completed outline so the student can fill in the details under major headings. As a variety, provide the details and have students fill in headings.

- **Remove neatness** as a grading criteria.

- Design assignments to be **evaluated** on specific parts of the writing process (prioritization).

- **Reduce copying** aspects of tasks, such as providing a math worksheet rather than requiring the student to copy problems from the book. A *copying buddy* can be helpful in copying the problems using carbon paper.

- Have younger students use large **graph paper** for math calculations to keep columns and rows straight. Older students may use loose leaf paper turned sideways to help maintain straight columns.

- Allow and encourage the use of **abbreviations** for in-class writing assignments (such as *b/4* for *before* or *b/c* for *because*). Have the student keep a list of appropriate abbreviations in his notebook and taped to his desk for easy reference. Begin with only a few and increase as the first few become automatic.

- Reinforce the **positive** aspects of the student's efforts.

- Be **patient**.

- **Encourage** the student to be patient with herself.

Chapter 13

Written Expression

Writing is easy. Just put down one word after another and drop in a comma when you want to slow down and a period when you want to stop. Make sure every sentence has a subject and a verb, preferably in that order, and sprinkle in a few adjectives and adverbs just to liven things up. (Lederer 1995, 1)

While some students may express these sentiments about writing, many other students agonize over the process of writing. Writing is not an easy process, but one that requires preplanning and organization. This process can be particularly cumbersome for the student with dyslexia or dysgraphia.

The process of writing creates excessive demands on active working memory because of the multiple steps which need to be performed simultaneously. Writing requires thought and knowledge of the subject. It also requires automatic letter form and an understanding of the mechanics for putting together sentences, using accurate grammar, punctuation, syntax, and spelling. Mel Levine has described the writing process as a major juggling act, where the writer must simultaneously juggle a wide range of components. When any one of these subtasks is difficult, the student struggles even more to focus on the other components. (Levine 1998)

Many students do not understand that writing is a *process* and not merely a task to be performed in one step. Young students need to begin to develop their understanding of the writing process as early as possible. The basic skills at these early levels are to generate information, elaborate and explain the information, and create sentences in a logical order. The student also needs to understand how to write for different readers and different purposes. This will help him utilize appropriate skills to make sure his writing will be understood by the reader. This particular aspect can be a significant problem for students whose oral language may not always be clear, well-developed, and easily understood. The conundrum occurs when this aspect is a significant problem for those students whose oral language is clear and well-developed.

When many students are presented with a basic writing assignment, they are able to consider the question, compile information, and then explain their ideas in writing. This type of assignment is in reality a compilation of a number of smaller language-based steps. The dyslexic or dysgraphic student needs to work on each one of these steps very explicitly, with substantial spiraling, exposure, and practice on each specific step. In so doing, the student can eventually learn to apply the steps independently. It is critical to realize that this is not a process learned by osmosis; students need to be explicitly taught key subtasks for pre-writing and writing. The basic pre-writing subtasks are comprehension, metacognitive awareness, staging, gathering and developing ideas, rehearsal, and organization. The basic writing subtasks are drafting, proofreading, editing, multiple drafts, proofing, and editing, and then final writing.

The Pre-writing Subtasks

Comprehension

Students must *comprehend* the vocabulary used in instructions, the nature of the writing task, the concepts, and the content. Many older students do well to maintain a writing notebook (or a special location within their loose-leaf binder) with a list of key words and their meanings. To use such a list, students need to be taught explicitly and exactly what each word means, with substantial discussion, clarification, modeling, and practice. Six of the most common key words are *apply, analyze, evaluate, recall, synthesize*, and *understand*, which are presented and explained in Figure 13.1 on the next page. Additional key words are listed on the chart on page 260.

Metacognitive Awareness

Metacognitive awareness helps students focus on the nature and purpose of writing. While this is vital for all students, it is absolutely essential for the student with dyslexia or dysgraphia. Students need to be taught to ask themselves key questions during each step in the writing process. Such questions will allow them to eventually be independent in developing their finished product. The habit of asking oneself relevant questions is essential because many learning disabled students lack the automatic ability to self-question and plan effectively, and they need specific, explicit, directed instruction to learn to do this. Students with language-based learning disabilities often lack the language structures to perform the self-talk on their own without explicit modeling. At the very least, they need to ask themselves, "Am I being clear? Have I answered the question and/or addressed the topic?" The presence or lack of metacognitive awareness often differentiates the dyslexic student who is successful in college from the dyslexic who is not.

Figure 13.1—Key words for thinking and writing.

If you are asked to . . .	You should be ready to . . .
Apply	**Use what you've learned** • to select the most important details • to organize information • to show how something works • to diagram or draw an example
Analyze	**Examine material closely to understand it better** • by making connections between this and other ideas • by studying cause and effect • by carefully explaining • by explaining similarities and differences among two or more items
Evaluate	**Judge the worth of the material** • by pointing out its strengths and weaknesses • by giving your opinions • by convincing someone else
Recall	**Remember what you've learned** • by listing important details • by defining terms • by clustering information
Synthesize	**Reshape material into a new form** • by inventing a better way of doing something • by predicting what will happen next • by creating something similar
Understand	**Show that you understand what you've learned** • by giving examples • by explaining how something works

Following are some sample metacognitive questions for students to use during the brainstorming process and for self-talk while writing:
- Who am I writing for? (Who is my audience?)
- What is the best way to address my audience?
- Why am I writing this?
- What do I already know about this topic?

- Can I relate this topic to anything I already know?
- How can I group my ideas?
- What is my topic?
- Have I answered the question?
- Have I addressed the topic?
- Do I know related topics?
- Where can I get more information?
- What is the best way to present this information?

The student's level of critical thinking skills must also be considered because often students with learning differences lag behind their peers in development of higher order, abstract skills. Teachers need to be aware of how realistic their assumptions are regarding a student's abstract thinking skills for given assignments, especially with the wide range of development that will occur in the middle and high school years.

As students begin to organize their information, they can ask themselves additional questions such as:
- Can I organize my ideas according to a text structure that I know?
- What do I think is the most important thing about my ideas?
- What new words have I learned?
- What new things did I learn?
- Is there something I still don't understand?
- What do I still want to know?
- Am I being clear?
- Have I tried my best?

Staging
In helping students appreciate that writing is a process, the concept of staging is very important. Staging is analyzing the task into its subcomponents, sequencing the subtasks appropriately, and then performing each one independently prior to integrating and pulling them together. Each one of the steps within the writing process needs to be explicitly taught. Substantial modeling, spiraling, and practice are necessary before most students are able to independently analyze a task into its subcomponents. This skill is useful for all students, but especially critical for the dyslexic and dysgraphic student.

Initially, staging can be used as part of the assignment, as in the following examples:
- For this paragraph, I want you to focus on using descriptive words.
- For this essay, we will not worry about punctuation or spelling, but focus on the clarity of the message.

- For this assignment, I want you to focus on how you begin your sentences. Use at least four different types of sentence beginnings.

By staging activities this way, teachers can help students focus on particular components. As they develop their own style and process of writing, they will then learn to use staging more independently. As they write, they should be encouraged to focus on one key aspect at a time. It is important to emphasize to students and help them realize that writing is a process that requires more than one quick draft.

With long-term writing activities, it is critical to allow enough time for good spacing between the stages. It is very hard for a student to edit or proofread something very soon after writing it. Dyslexics, especially, may read what they intended, rather than what they actually wrote. In contrast, it can be relatively interesting to proofread a passage several days or a week later, and the task becomes more satisfying because it is easier to improve one's writing. This type of approach requires that students avoid doing their assignments at the last minute. Consequently, it is imperative to help them identify the sub-tasks that need to be done and provide a time line for completion of each sub-task, with the time line allowing sufficient resting time between various drafts. Teachers will need to evaluate, support, model for, and encourage students at each stage. The editing aspect of the writing task is critical for all students, but especially for students who learn differently.

Gathering and Developing Ideas

To help students in the gathering of information stage, a simple KWL chart is useful. KWL stands for *know, want, learn*. As students research information, they can set up the KWL chart to help them organize the information they gather. There are three columns in the chart. The first two columns are filled in before the gathering of information takes place. The last column is filled in during and after the gathering of information. Figure 13.2 provides an example of the KWL chart. A full-size chart is provided on page 251.

Figure 13.2—KWL chart

Topic:		
Source(s):		
What do I know?	What do I want to learn?	What did I learn?

This is a good point in the process to work as a group and to pull in a large variety of strategies, using different modes, modalities, and multisensory activities. The variety helps stimulate interest and excitement in the task and leads to more creative brainstorming. When brainstorming occurs as a group process, the students' ideas feed upon and encourage each other. Use of visual organizers combined with the brainstorming process helps utilize the visual processing strengths of many of the students.

There are so many activities that can be used to stimulate brainstorming, as a teacher's creativity is boundless. Examples of just a few ideas that can be used follow:

- **Camera-head game:** Have students look at a portion of the room for 10 seconds, then close their eyes and recall all they can. They then open their eyes and notice what they missed. The process is repeated, helping the students understand that they are taking a picture with their mind and that they should focus on details.

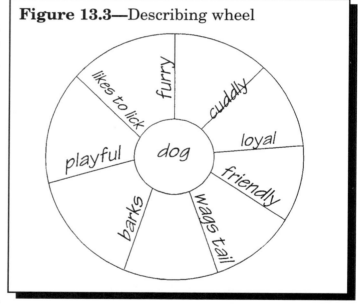

Figure 13.3—Describing wheel

- **Visualization:** Read the students a descriptive passage. Have them close their eyes and visualize as you are reading. Their visualizations can be guided with specific questions, such as "What color do you imagine the boy's shirt to be?" Afterwards, have them draw their visualizations, and then discuss the variations.

- **Storyboards:** Have students draw out or map out a sequence of events using successive squares on a piece of paper.

- **Pantomiming, charades, mimes:** Act out the information or story.

- **Describing wheel:** A describing wheel helps describe a subject or an object. The main topic is written in the middle of the wheel and words that describe the topic are written on the spokes. Encourage students to use the five senses in describing their topic. In the example of a dog in Figure 13.3, *bark* evokes the auditory sense; *licks, furry,* and *cuddly* suggest the tactile, kinesthetic sense; and *wags tail* encourages a visual image.

Rehearsal

Rehearsal and discussion before writing is critical. There is an important link between discussing a topic and writing a topic, and generally it is easier for students to talk through the topic prior to beginning to write it. This is especially true with younger students, but is also very helpful, although often omitted, for older students. Sufficient pre-organizational activities prior to the writing activity is a habit that should be strongly developed.

The point of oral rehearsal is to make connections among bits of information students already know. Students can then pull this information together with graphic organizers to help organize the task and move it from an oral task to a writing task. Generally, as students become older, oral rehearsal is neglected. However, it is important, even for students in middle school and high school. Without connections between different aspects of the task, students' writing will not be as clear, strong, or analytical as might be possible otherwise. Discussion also helps clarify disorganized ideas. In a discussion format, students can be encouraged and led through clarification. Students should continually be encouraged to ask questions, as this is a habit that they can use to clarify their writing. Encourage them to ask questions about what they read, what they hear, and even what they see. Students should look at all sides of a question and support their thoughts with good reasons, examples, and facts.

If students think they know *what* something is, they should then ask:
- Why?
- When?
- How?
- How much?
- Why not?

To encourage students to move past the concrete and use more analytical and inferential thinking, they can play the "What's Missing?" game. Begin with a simple picture, such as a woman and a man holding a baby. Cover the picture of the baby and ask students, "What's missing?" As they guess, ask them to identify which cues in the picture led them to their conclusion, and then explain why that cue led to their conclusion.

The best types of pictures to use at the beginning are those that provide obvious cues. For example:

- a family around a table in a kitchen or dining room. Cover up the food on the table.

- a woods or garden containing a large tree. Cover the entire tree except the trunk.

As the students progress, cover up a more subtle part of the picture.

Organization

Effective writing is absolutely dependent on good organization skills, and the aspect of organization is critical for students who learn differently. Students need to know how to organize sentences within a paragraph and paragraphs within a passage. They also need to know how to present details in a logical fashion and with good clarity. Essay writing is more complex than creative writing, as students need to integrate the organization of the information around development of a thesis. Generally, students who struggle to sort and organize language-based information will also struggle with clarity, conciseness, and effectiveness of writing assignments. Therefore, it is important that these students understand how to structure different types of tasks for different purposes. Concrete visual techniques are extremely helpful, such as prewriting worksheets and visual organizers. Organization should be very thorough, specific, and well taught, and may, in essence, be the most critical aspect of the writing process for dyslexic and dysgraphic students. It is a step which addresses the organizational deficits so commonly found in these students.

Organizing the format is a critical step for students. They first need to decide on the topic and purpose for the writing assignment. A prewriting worksheet is useful, and you'll find one to use with your students on page 252. (Reed 1995)

Visual organization strategies are effective methods that provide a concrete alternative to traditional outlining. Such strategies allow students to organize material in a visual pattern so they can see the relationships among the information. It allows them to represent connections more easily and promotes fluency, flexibility, and more originality. However, with the inclusion of many outlining programs within word processing computer software, the process of outlining has been greatly facilitated for students. Efficient outline programs are available in most newer versions of word processing programs, as well as in the software program *Inspiration*®. This latter program is exciting for many because it automatically converts between a mind map and outline format.

Prior to deciding what type of organizer to use, students need to determine the purpose of their writing. With the younger students, simple terms to describe the types of writing are useful. As the students mature, the descriptions of the types of writing can consequently become more mature. The four basic types of paragraphs (and ultimately multi-paragraph writings) include:

- **Descriptive:** A descriptive paragraph describes something.

- **Narrative:** A narrative paragraph tells a story.
- **Persuasive:** A persuasive paragraph supports an opinion.
- **Expository:** An expository paragraph explains something.

Expository paragraphs are very important and often create a difficult challenge for students. These types of paragraphs may explain ideas, give directions, or show how to do something. It is important for students to recognize that an expository paragraph must use transition words, such as *first* and *second* or *most importantly*. Because of the organizational difficulties of many students who learn differently, it is critical that they organize their facts and sequence them appropriately before beginning to write this type of paragraph. Developing expository skills is critical for use throughout one's school career, as well as in many workplace situations.

Organizing the ideas may be a lengthy step for the students, but as this subtask becomes more automatic, the students will begin to appreciate its usefulness. To help students begin to think and plan systematically, the task should be made as concrete as possible. This is the value of visual or graphic organizers—they organize the information concretely and visually. The style of the organizer depends upon the nature of the task. Some of the many styles are presented on the handouts on pages 253-256 and have been referenced by a large number of authors. (Pehrrson and Robinson 1985; Pehrrson and Denner 1989; Margulies 1991; Richards 1993; Tarricone 1995)

Outlines and graphic organizers for multi-paragraph and essay writing are constructed in a similar fashion to a graphic organizer for paragraphs. Many students may want to have one overall organizer (with thesis statement, body, and conclusion) as well as individual organizers for each component. Some students prefer mapping while others prefer outlining. It is important for students to have a variety of tools to match the strategy to the task and so they can feel comfortable with the strategy they choose.

The Writing Subtasks

Drafting

The concept of a draft is often very foreign for learning disabled students, as many tend to think their first draft is also their final paper. Or, they wish it to be so because of all the effort required to produce the draft. It is important for students to learn how to use organizers to generate an efficient draft and to realize that the draft is just one part of the process.

Prior to starting the actual writing of the draft, it is very useful to encourage students to brainstorm some of the more difficult words they may want to use.

They should make a list of these words, spelling them phonetically and checking the spelling with an electronic spell checker or the spell checker in a word processing program. They can use this as a reference for at least some of the more difficult words they will use and the flow of their thoughts will be less impaired by potential spelling difficulties. This will also encourage them to use more sophisticated words, rather than restricting their word usage to simple, easy-to-spell words.

Many students need to begin their focus on writing with the concept of a topic sentence. A graphic analogy can be to compare the topic sentence to the engine on a train. This sentence is the main idea that connects all other sentences and pulls them along, just as the engine pulls along the cars of the train. Generally, a paragraph begins with a topic sentence to tell the reader what the paragraph is about. The topic sentence has two main parts:

- The subject: the subject of a topic sentence has to be specific enough to explain in one paragraph.

- The focus: the focus is usually a feeling or an attitude about the subject and it lets the reader know what the writer is going to say on the topic.

Proofreading

Proofreading skills are critical for all students, but most importantly for students who have some language-based difficulty. Proofing involves reflecting upon what is written and analyzing the mechanics, structure, and organization. Editing involves reflecting on what is written with an eye toward making it clearer, more persuasive, stronger, or more descriptive.

The concept of staging is critical during the process of proofreading. A useful strategy is to teach students the acronym COPS. (Schumaker, Nolan, and Deshler 1985) This encourages the student to proofread four times, once for each of the following components: **C**apitalization, **O**rganization, **P**unctuation, and **S**pelling. This does not guarantee that the student will not make mistakes in these areas, nor does it guarantee that the student will find all mistakes. However, the process does help the student attend to the critical elements in a way that may compensate for gaps in active working memory. Each element must be defined specifically for the students depending on their writing level, age, and overall linguistic development. Figures 13.4a and 13.4b present graphic representations to accompany COPS. (Richards 1993, 74-79)

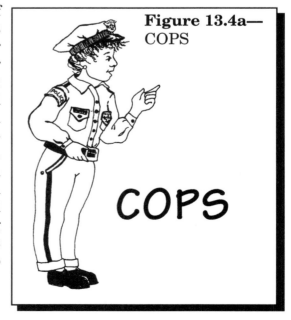

Figure 13.4a—
COPS

COPS

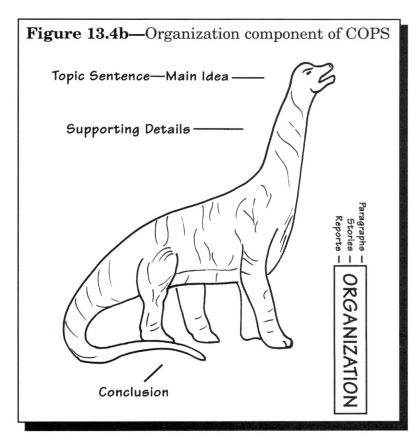

Figure 13.4b—Organization component of COPS

Topic Sentence—Main Idea

Supporting Details

Paragraphs
Stories
Reports

ORGANIZATION

Conclusion

Other valuable formats for students may include checklists or self-evaluation forms. The 10 Item Proofreading Checklist on page 257 (adapted from Reed 1995) and the Proofreading Self-Evaluation on page 258 (adapted from Reed 1995) are two examples that are easy to use. The use of a self-evaluation form is particularly valuable in increasing metacognitive awareness.

Editing
Editing is a more advanced process than proofreading and is dependent on strong metacognitive skills. This step helps students be aware of the reasons for their writing and it requires them to ask themselves questions as they move through the editing process. At the beginning, students can be asked to check that they have the three main parts in their writing: the beginning, the middle, and the end. A simplified way to explain these three parts follows:

- The *beginning* should name the subject in an interesting way.
- The *middle* should tell about the subject.
- The *ending* should say something important about the subject.

It is also useful to help students develop a list of some of the favorite ways they can "hook" readers into their writing in the first paragraph. An important hook will set the tone and pull the reader into the paragraph. Some more advanced examples for hooking a reader in the beginning of an essay are to use one of the following:

- A quote or dialogue
- A startling fact or anecdote
- An action or description
- An opinion

Students can ask themselves questions regarding their introductory paragraph (or their introductory sentence in a single-paragraph essay) to increase their metacognitive awareness. Four relevant questions are as follows:

- Will the introduction arouse the interest of my reader?
- Does the introduction direct my reader's attention from a broad, general idea to a more specific thesis or idea?
- Does the introduction limit the topic and focus the central idea?
- Does the introduction establish a relationship between me, the writer, and my reader?

Transition and linking words are very critical and many students have difficulty using words other than *and*. Some students may write a paragraph wherein each sentence starts the same way. It is useful to help these students learn to use different types of transition or linking words. The chart on page 259 lists transition and linking words in a variety of categories. Students can be given an assignment requiring them to use, for example, three different transition words in their paragraph.

Conclusions are also a very difficult aspect for many dyslexic students. They have trouble organizing the language information and pulling it together toward a cohesive ending. Some helpful questions to ask about a conclusion for a paragraph or essay are:

- Does my conclusion tie in smoothly with the body?
- Does my conclusion summarize the main arguments?
- Does my conclusion remind the reader of the basic theme?
- Is my ending striking enough to leave a lasting impression?
- Does my ending maintain a tone consistent with the rest of the essay?

As students advance, they can extend their editing checklist with questions such as the following:

- Did I focus on a certain part of my subject instead of trying to say everything about it?
- Do I need to add any information, details, or explanations?
- Do I need to cut any unnecessary information that is not supportive to my main idea?
- Do I need to rewrite any parts to increase the clarity of my explanation?
- Do I need to reorder any parts of my writing? Is my method of organization effective?

You will find additional metacognitive questions in Figure 13.5 on page 243. (Tarricone 1995, 36)

Figure 13.5—Metacognitive questions

Some metacognitive questions to use during editing are:
- Did I answer the question asked?
- Did I explain it in a clear manner?
- Can my reader understand my main point?
- Did I use key words?
- Did I use transitional words?
- What part should I make clearer?
- What questions might my reader have?
- Did I use an effective text structure? (organization)
- Is it interesting?
- What parts do I like best?
- What could I do to make it more interesting?
- Did I use appropriate examples to illustrate my points?
- Did I support my viewpoints?

Multiple Drafts, Proofing, Editing

Students may need to repeat the drafting, proofing, and editing steps more than once or twice. This depends primarily on the complexity of the content, but also on the student's skill level. Use of a word processor on a computer facilitates proofing and editing and makes the concept of multiple drafts more palatable, since students can then avoid rewriting each draft.

Final Writing

This step requires the students to incorporate revisions from the proofreading and editing stages with emphasis on accurate inclusion of corrections and suggestions. Many times, students will have difficulty understanding how each step is linked and they have trouble applying and including their revised ideas into their final drafts. These students will need extra help through modeling, explanations, and practice. At this step, additional emphasis is placed on the neatness and overall presentation of the writing, ideally incorporated with word processing skills.

Reinforcement Activities

Subject/Verb Agreement

Many students with language-based learning difficulties do not automatically recognize errors in subject/verb agreement, especially in lengthier sentences, and most especially when they have written the sentences themselves. One strategy to help students learn to proofread their papers for these types of errors involves the following steps:

- Make sure they understand and can identify nouns and verbs.
- Teach firm identification of prepositions through multisensory strategies.
- Teach the student to mark all prepositional phrases within a lengthy sentence.
- Teach the student to recognize the subject and its corresponding verb, using the unmarked phrases.

A concrete multisensory strategy to help students identify prepositions is to utilize wads of cotton and a toy airplane. Using a small plastic airplane or a paper model of an airplane, the plane can be used to demonstrate prepositions in relation to the cloud (represented by the cotton). Any relationship that the plane can exhibit with the cotton is generally a preposition: *below* the cloud, *behind* the cloud, *in front of* the cloud, *through* the cloud, *beneath* the cloud, *toward* the cloud, *under* the cloud, and *over* the cloud, as in Figure 13.6.

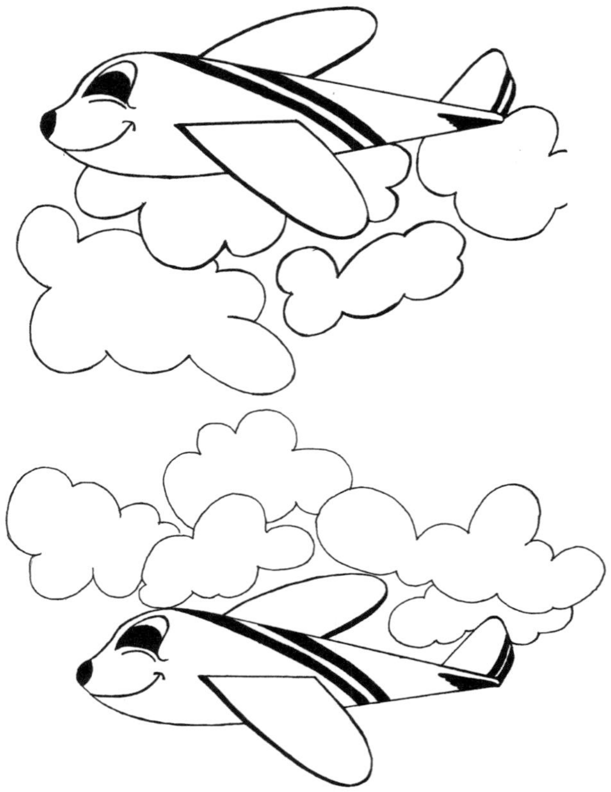

It is important that students understand that a preposition shows the relationship between the noun or pronoun which follows it and some other words in the sentence. Using the airplane as an example, students can recognize that a preposition is a word that points or shows location. The word *of* needs to be given special consideration.

Following is an example of a long sentence given to a fourth grade student to help her identify subject/verb agreement.

Figure 13.6—Teaching prepositions: *over* the cloud and *under* the cloud

"Another Merry Little Breeze, up on the Crooked Little Path on the hill, spied the hind legs of a fat beetle sticking out from under a flat stone." (Burgess 1985, 128)

The steps followed by the student are as follows:
- The student identifies the prepositions: *upon, on, of, from*
- The student then marks the corresponding prepositional phrases:
  up on the Crooked Little Path
  on the hill
  of a fat beetle
  from under a flat stone
- The remaining unmarked words are:
  Another Merry Little Breeze
  spied
  sticking
- The student then identifies the noun that is the subject (*Merry Little Breeze*) and the related verb (*spied*) and determines that both are in singular format.

Enhancing Vocabulary Usage

One of the ways to help students enhance the sophistication and efficiency of their written expression is to help them learn to use vocabulary words with greater variety and flexibility. Vocabulary development is critical, not only for concept development, but also for clarifying points of information. A more extensive vocabulary usage also enhances critical thinking. Dyslexics learn vocabulary more efficiently through multisensory means. They rarely retain meaning of new words by merely looking them up in a dictionary. A variety of activities can be used, including miming, charades, artwork, mind maps, and visualization

Visualization

Use of imagery helps pull in metacognitive skills, visual spatial skills, and often some awareness of body movements. This is because imagery can involve more than just visual imagery, but also an image of muscle movements, smells, tastes, or sensations (such as the wind blowing). Therefore, it is very valuable to use visualization in helping students to enhance their analysis of a situation as well as their use of words to verbalize and describe the images in their visualization.

Students can begin to enhance their visualization skills by using descriptions of a common object. Food is usually a good object to start with because it can be eaten afterward. Students can work in pairs or small groups and, using real fruit such as a strawberry, answer questions about the shape, weight, color, texture, seeds, moisture, size, sweetness, etc. One student in each group closes his eyes and imagines the strawberry. Another student asks what his strawberry looks like, what it weighs, or how he imagines it tastes. Students can also imagine what it would be like to be that fruit and change from a blossom into a newly formed berry. Other scenarios could include:

- being picked off the stem
- having bugs crawling on you
- feeling the sun on you
- feeling the rain on you
- getting cold at night
- being smelled and admired by someone
- being on a plate
- being examined and having the leaves plucked off

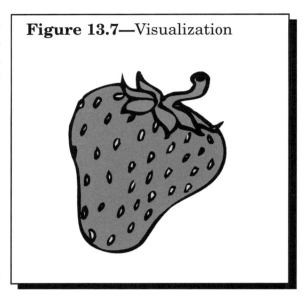

Figure 13.7—Visualization

Visualization can also begin with a simple picture (Figure 13.7) and move to more complex pictures, or the input can be purely auditory. It is good to use a variety of techniques for variability. Nanci Bell, in *Visualizing and Verbalizing for Language Comprehension and Thinking*, presents a very structured, systematic approach, moving from visualizing pictures through visualizing for comprehension of a whole chapter. (Bell 1991) She uses structure words to provide a guide for including detail in the verbalization and visualization, using *what, size, color, number, shape*, as well as more precise words such as *movement, mood, background, perspective, when*, and *sound*.

Laura Rose also has visualization activities wherein she links the visualization with reading comprehension. Students are read a passage or a story and then asked very specific questions (Rose 1989; Rose 1991) relating to setting, characters, weather, colors, thoughts, time of day, period of the story, or predictions. For example,

- Characters: *How old is the boy? How is he dressed?*
- Weather: *What does the sky look like?*
- Thoughts: *What do you suppose the boy is thinking?*
- Period of story: *Is this happening in modern times or some other time?*
- Predictions: *Do you think he will . . . ? What will happen next?*

Understanding Words Used in Directions

Many times, students may feel they understand directions, but in reality they do not have a full understanding of the primary instructional word or words. This can obviously create difficulties in how they perform the assignment. It is important to spend substantial time with practice, explanations, demonstrations, and a wide variety of activities to make sure students easily recognize the meanings behind the primary key words used in giving instructions—especially essay questions.

Page 260 provides key words beyond the six most common in Figure 13.1 that students need to comprehend for writing. (Kemper 1995, 307) These also enhance their ability to think about and analyze information.

Confusable Words

Homonyms, including both homophones and homographs as well as words that are phonetically similar, are often confused in students' writing. It is important for students to understand many of these more common word pairs (or triads) and also to have a readily accessible reference list of these words. The meaning of these words can be analyzed and manipulated through a variety of activities, including miming, charades, dramatization, and artwork, as suggested in the section on vocabulary. Mnemonics are also of great help to solidify the differences between important word pairs. Page 261 is a reference list of 24 of the most common confusable word sets for elementary ages. (adapted from Kemper, Nathan, Sabranek 1996, 268-273)

Tom Swifty and Games

Tom Swift was a hero created by Edward Stratemeyer, wherein Tom and his peers never just said something; they always said it excitedly or sadly or hurriedly. (Lederer 1988, 73) Tom Swifty games use puns to vary the adverbs in statements.

The benefits of playing such games are many. Students have fun with words while they play with word meaning, extend their vocabularies, and learn the expressive value of vivid adverbs. Some Tom Swifty examples include:

- "I love pancakes," said Tom flippantly.
- "My pants are wrinkled," said Tom ironically.
- "I hate pineapples," said Tom dolefully.
- "Let's go to McDonald's®," said Tom archly.
- "I'll have the dark bread," said Tom wryly.
- "Look at those newborn kittens," said Tom literally.
- "I've lost my flowers," said Tom lackadaisically.

Older students enjoy playing Tom Swifty games. The activity can begin as multiple choice wherein the teacher provides the phrase and then a selection of adverbs, an example of which is shown in Figure 13.8 on page 248. As the students progress, they can create their own complete phrases without the cues.

Use of an electronic, hand-held reference tool is often very helpful in finding adverbs for a Tom Swifty game. For example, using a Franklin Language Master® and given the phrase "I love eating crow," the student can first look up a synonym for crow. Selecting the synonym *raven*, they can punch in *raven* with a

Figure 13.8—Tom Swifty game

	said Tom . . .
1. "I must attend my flock"	a) grossly
2. "My pencil is dull"	b) trenchantly
3. "That makes 144"	c) moodily
4. "She tore my valentine in two"	d) sheepishly
5. "I'm a ditch digger"	e) pridefully
6. "I'm a lion hunter"	f) delightfully
7. "Whoops, another power failure"	g) pointlessly
8. "I milk cows"	h) halfheartedly

Answers: 1-d, 2-g, 3-a, 4-h, 5-b, 6-e, 7-f, 8-c

wild card and the electronic spell checker will give the word *ravenously*. They can then double-check the meaning to see what the new word means and create the sentence, "I love eating crow," said Tom ravenously.

Related to Tom Swifty games are the Croaker games. In Croakers, the verb rather than the adverb supplies the pun. Some examples follow:

- "My pet frog died," Tom croaked.
- "I love cats," Tom mused.
- "I love beagles," Tom dogmatized.
- "I used to be a miner," Tom exclaimed.
- "I feel empty inside," Tom hollered.

To help guide students in developing creative Croakers, the following sample dialogue can be used.

Teacher:	Finish this Croaker: "I hate sweet potatoes," Tom _____
Student:	Tom potatoed.
Teacher:	Does that make sense?
Student:	No. How about "Tom said sweetly?"
Teacher:	That's good. But can you think of one word that would fit? What's another word for "sweet potatoes?"
Student:	Yams.
Teacher:	Can you think of a verb that uses the word *yam* within it?
Student:	Yammered! "I hate sweet potatoes," Tom yammered.

As students become more skilled in these types of semantic manipulations, the double croaker can be used, in which both the verb and the adverb or the verb and the noun are coordinated to provide the pun within the sentence.

Some examples include:

- "Where did you get that meat?" Tom bridled hoarsely.
- "This meat is hard to chew," Tom beefed jerkily.
- "I train big cats," Tom lionized categorically.
- "I hate reading Victor Hugo," said Les miserably.

May you and your students enjoy many creative, fun, and meaningful writing experiences. The more fun students have, the more they practice.

Sample Activity

Activity: **State Unit**

This activity describes a sequence of a variety of activities used with a group of third to fifth grade dyslexic students, many of whom are also dysgraphic. The unit, performed over an extended period of time, exemplifies a sequence that can be used to incorporate many of the techniques discussed. Students work in groups, with each group focusing on a specific state.

Step 1: Gather information

In this step, students write letters to various agencies in their state, watch videos about their state, sing songs, and read and role play stories to gather information. They use a KWL Chart (found on page 251) to keep track of their ideas.

Step 2: Diorama

Students decide on the important information about their state, which greatly helps enhance their skills in saliency determination. They represent that information in a diorama, with each group deciding on its own type of construction materials. This step helps enhance students' skills in saliency determination.

Step 3: Creation of mind map

Students use the information collected for the diorama to create a mind map on paper. In their discussion, they categorize information, organize information, and select the main points for each section in their state report. They use a Franklin Language Master® to help facilitate spelling as needed. Some groups use the Inspiration® program on the computer.

Step 4: First draft writing

Students use their mind map to generate a first draft. Since this is a group project, different students are responsible for different components of the report. Depending upon the students' skill levels and writing proficiency, they use techniques such as dictating, writing with a pen, or typing on a computer.

Step 5: Organizing the report

The students pull their paragraphs together and proofread the whole report for general flow, content, and transitions. They decide upon some changes related to organizing, sequencing, and integrating the material.

Step 6: Proofing

Step 7: Editing

Step 8: Group presentations

The students decide on the main parts of their report to present to the rest of the class. They are allowed (and encouraged) to create songs, perform a skit, create a model or painting, pull in sections of videos, or use whatever modality they desire to represent their state.

Step 9: Interstate Fair Day

Students set up a display to explain their state, selecting music, food, and related activities. Students visit each others' booths using a Passport, with the goal of having their Passport stamped in each state. Parents are invited to visit the Fair.

Topic:		
Source(s):		
What do I know?	What do I want to learn?	What did I learn?

Prewriting Worksheet

Topic:

What do I know? _____

Narrow to a specific aspect of the subject _____

Narrow again _____

Purpose:

My intention _____

The effect I want to have on my audience _____

Audience:

Who my audience is _____

Their special characteristics _____

Attitude:

How do I feel about my topic? _____

How will my attitude affect the tone of my writing? _____

_____

Experience:

What I know about this subject _____

_____

What other information I need _____

_____

Where I will get more information _____

_____

Persona:

The role/approach I should take
toward my audience: I am   ___ an equal   ___ an authority   ___ a character

Mode:

The form of writing that is
best for me: ___ essay   ___ story   ___ letter   ___ poem

I will use: ___ narration   ___ description   ___ time order   ___ step order

___ example   ___ cause-effect   ___ compare-contrast

Sequential and Chronological maps

These are used to help students organize information over time or to explain a process. They can deal with years, eras, periods, steps, or stages.

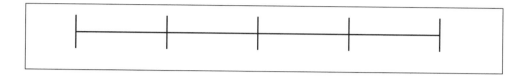

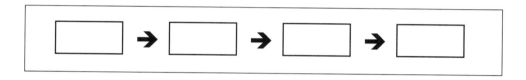

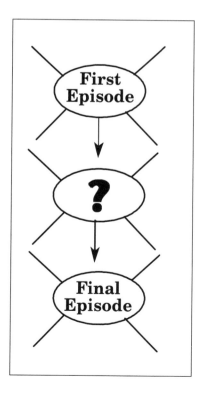

details	details	details	details

Descriptive maps

Descriptive maps help students list or explain reasons. They can also be used for categorization as well as to describe characteristics and attributes.

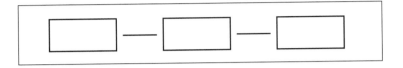

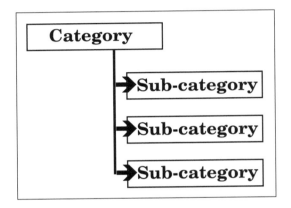

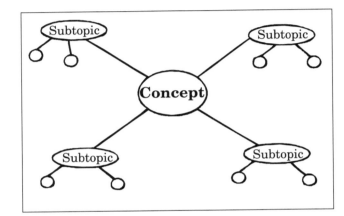

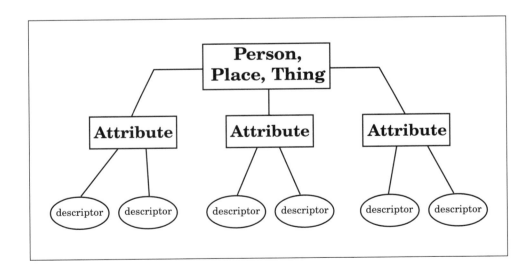

Compare and Contrast maps

These maps help students discover and analyze similarities and differences. They also help highlight specific attributes which need to be compared. They simultaneously help students see the "big picture" as well as the details

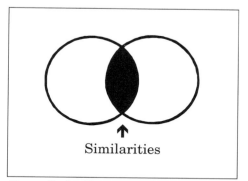

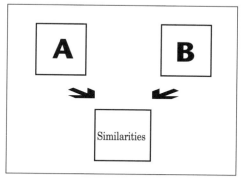

Also called a Venn Diagram.

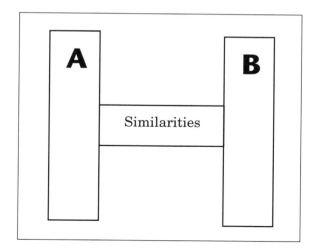

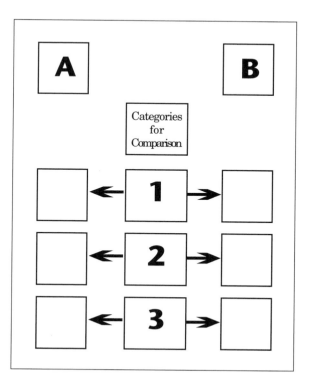

Cause and Effect maps

Many times, it is important to indicate one or more cause or one or more effect, and this can be done through this form of organizer. Related compositions often use words like *result, because*, and *therefore*.

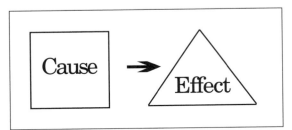

Figure 13.8a

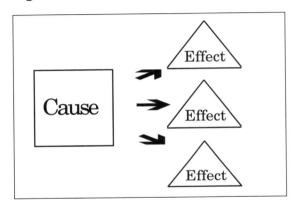

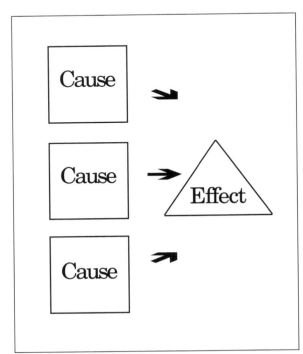

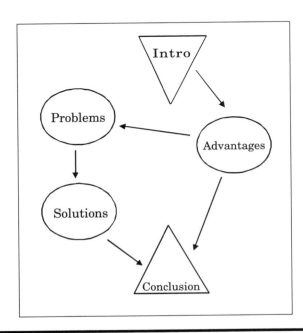

Proofreading Checklist

____ 1. Make sure that all sentences are complete.

____ 2. Change run-on sentences to two or more sentences.

____ 3. Check for omitted words or word endings.

____ 4. Make sure that action words (verbs) have correct endings. Check the nouns and pronouns that are the subject of the action.

____ 5. Check capital letters:
- ✔ First word in a sentence
- ✔ First letter of a proper name: people, pets, places, holidays, days, months, abbreviations such as *Ave., St., Mrs., Mr.*
- ✔ The word *I*
- ✔ The important words of titles

____ 6. Check final punctuation or sentences:
- ✔ Period at the end of a statement
- ✔ Questions mark if a sentence is a question and needs an answer
- ✔ Exclamation mark if the sentence shows a strong emotion (fear, anger, excitement)

____ 7. Check other punctuation:
- ✔ Quotation marks, commas, etc., in quotations
- ✔ Commas with words in a series
- ✔ Commas after introductory clauses
- ✔ Commas between two independent clauses joined by a conjunction
- ✔ Apostrophes in contractions and possessive nouns

____ 8. Check for misspelled words. Look up the word(s) if you are not sure.

____ 9. Check for homonyms such as *there / their / they're* and *to / two / too.*

___ 10. Recheck to make sure you found everything and, if possible, have someone else proofread too.

Proofreading Self-Evaluation

1. **Answer the following questions by placing a check in the most appropriate box.**

	Yes	No	Somewhat
a) Have I fulfilled the assignment?	❑	❑	❑
b) Have I stuck to the topic?	❑	❑	❑
c) Is my writing organized and easy to understand?	❑	❑	❑
d) Have I supported my statements with details and reasons?	❑	❑	❑
e) Have I kept unimportant and unrelated information out of my writing?	❑	❑	❑

2. **Refer to items a) through e) in #1.**
   a) Which is my strongest area? (Put a happy face next to it.)
   b) Which is my weakest area? (Put a sad face next to it.)

3. **Check the most appropriate box.**

	Yes	No
a) Have I used interesting, descriptive words?	❑	❑
b) Have I written any sentence fragments or run-ons?	❑	❑
c) Have I used various types of sentences?	❑	❑
d) Have I put capital letters where they are needed?	❑	❑
e) Have I used punctuation marks correctly?	❑	❑

4. **Answer these questions on spelling and mechanics:**

	Good	Fair	Poor
a) My penmanship is	❑	❑	❑

   b) These are the letters I do not form as clearly as I could:

   _____

	Yes	No
c) Am I careful about my margins?	❑	❑
d) Am I careful not to place words too close to one another?	❑	❑
e) Do I indent my paragraphs?	❑	❑

   f) These are the words I use too often in my writing. They are sometimes repeated needlessly:

   _____

   _____

   g) I often misspelled these words:_____

   _____

5. Overall I am   ❑ very happy   ❑ satisfied   ❑ displeased with what I have written.

Transition or Linking Words

Words which can be used to show locations.

above	around	between	inside	outside
across	behind	by	into	over
against	below	down	near	throughout
along	beneath	in back of	off	to the right
among	beside	in front of	on top of	under

Words which can be used to show time.

about	during	until	yesterday	finally
after	first	meanwhile	next	then
at	second	today	soon	as soon as
before	third	tomorrow	later	when

Words which can be used to compare two things.

in the same way	likewise	as
similarly	like	also

Words which can be used to contrast things (show difference).

but	otherwise	still	even though
yet	on the other hand	although	

Words which can be used to emphasize a point.

again	for this reason	in fact

Words which can be used to add information.

again	and	for instance	as well
also	besides	next	along with
another	for example	finally	

Words which can be used to conclude or summarize.

as a result	finally	in conclusion	consequently
therefore	last	in summary	

Adapted from *Writer's Express*, (1995) by David Kemper, Ruth Nathan, & Patrick Sebranek

Key Words for Thinking and Writing

If you are asked to . . .	You should be ready to . . .
Compare	Cite similarities between two or more objects.
Contrast	Cite differences between two or more objects.
Compare and contrast	Look for both similarities and differences to show how two things are alike in several ways and to show how they are different.
Define	Tell about what the word or subject means, generally showing what the thing is and what it does.
Describe	Tell how something or someone looks, feels, or sounds. Use the five senses in describing.
Diagram	Provide a drawing, such as a mind map or a flow chart.
Discuss	Make sure your answer is analytical and has depth.
Explain	Tell how something happens or show how it works in a step-by-step fashion.
Illustrate	Use examples or provide a mind map or flow chart.
Interpret	Explain your own reasons and judgements and justify them using facts.
Justify	Provide logical reasons for your statements or conclusions and back these up with facts.
List	Include a variety of reasons, examples, and other details, generally in a list form.
Outline	Draft your answer using only the main points and supporting details, ideally using an outline form.
Prove	Present facts and details which show very clearly that something is true, ideally using a well-developed, logical argument.
Relate	Show the relationship or connection between ideas. Use an accompanying diagram if necessary.
Review	Write a critical summary to highlight main ideas, but also include your own judgements and opinions.
Summarize	Highlight main ideas without extensive proving of your analysis and opinions.
Trace	Explain the development, progress, history, or progression of an idea or concept.

Confusable Words

ant	aunt	An *ant* crawled onto my finger.	My *aunt* likes to tell jokes.
ate	eight	Liz *ate* lunch with me.	I have *eight* crayons.
bare	bear	My *bare* hands are freezing.	Ira has a teddy *bear*.
blew	blue	Eli *blew* the biggest bubble.	A robin's egg is *blue*.
dear	deer	My grandma is a *dear* woman.	The *deer* ran into the woods.
eye	I	Ellen winks her *eye*.	*I* love to draw dogs.
for	four	Miss Smith made cookies *for* us.	Suzy ate *four* tacos.
hear	here	I like to *hear* birds sing.	Who sits *here*?
knew	new	I *knew* my ABC's last year.	We have a *new* girl in our class.
know	no	Do you *know* her name?	Robert said, "*No*, I don't."
made	maid	We *made* popcorn for a snack.	Amelia Bedelia is a funny *maid*.
meat	meet	Some people don't eat *meat*.	I'll *meet* you at the clubhouse.
one	won	My baby brother is *one* year old.	Nancy *won* a prize in the contest.
read	red	Mr. Jones *read* a funny poem.	I gave him a *red* apple.
road	rode	The man lives on a country *road*.	He *rode* his bike to school.
sea	see	A *sea* is a body of water.	Come and *see* my pet snake.
sew	so	My grandma likes to *sew* for me.	I'll hurry *so* we're not late.
son	sun	My brother is my dad's *son*.	Plants need *sun* and water.
tail	tale	A beaver has a flat *tail*.	Cinderella is a fairy *tale*.

their	there	they're
	We used *their* bikes.	*There* are four of them.	*They're* mountain bikes.
	(*their* shows ownership)	(*There* is pointing)	(*they're* = they are)

to	two	too
	I like *to* read funny books.	I read *two* joke books today.	John likes joke books, *too*.

wear	where	I like to *wear* floppy hats.	*Where* are you going?
wood	would	The fence is made of *wood*.	Dawn *would* like to go home.
your	you're	What's *your* favorite video?	*You're* a great singer. (*you're* = you are)

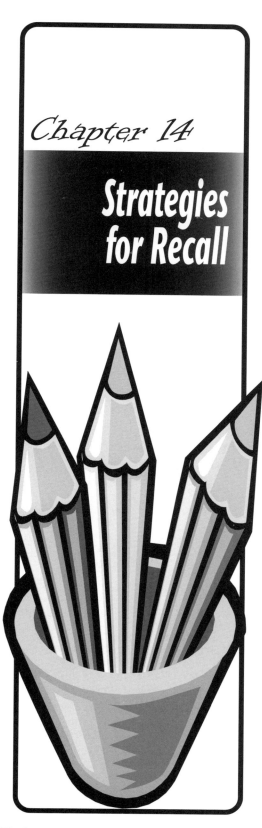

Chapter 14

Strategies for Recall

Dyslexics frequently have a very good ability to remember and analyze contextual information. However, many aspects of academic learning, especially rote sequential memory and associative memory, cause them substantial difficulty. These are the tasks that require students to remember a sequence (math facts, months of the year) or to relate two or more pieces of information, such as a name and a date. When students struggle, it is important for them to realize why the task is difficult (Is it the sequencing? Too many details?) and then develop an alternative strategy to deal with the difficulty.

Strategies provide a plan to help students remember information. Strategies pull in connections, bring in visual and other processing strengths, and help a student organize information, especially rote information, to remember and apply at a later time. Not all strategies work well for all students. Having a variety of tools to use will help each individual find a way to triumph over difficult tasks, as the tools help students pull in their strengths to compensate for their weaknesses. The charts on pages 289-290 provide a list of strategies which often benefit dyslexic learners by providing techniques that can be used within a wide range of learning situations. Often, more than one strategy can be pulled in. For example, many times visual mnemonics can be combined with imagery and perhaps even with music, using a rap or a simple song.

This chapter provides a few suggestions on using some of these strategies. The suggestions are a starting point for teachers, parents, and students to generate their own ideas regarding ways to add multisensory and connective techniques within a learning situation. The primary goals are to make information more concrete for the student, to increase retention and to facilitate understanding, and develop an ability to apply and use the information. These strategies all include the three S's—they are **s**tructured, **s**ystematic, and include **s**ensory input. Examples will be provided for use of imagery, mnemonics, mind mapping, metaphors, music, and rhythm.

Imagery

Helping students develop images enhances their engagement and interaction with the material. Images can be visual (imagining a picture or event), auditory (imagining a related sound or rhythm), kinesthetic (imagining a movement), or tactile (imagining the feel of something, such as a touch or the wind). Images that combine several factors are most effective and may be remembered the longest. Visualization begins to develop in very young children as they interact in a multisensory way with their environment. School age children are often not aware of their ability to visualize, but this skill can be developed and enhanced through structured practice.

Peg Word System

A popular mnemonic system that uses visualization is the *peg word system*. Key words are established to serve as pegs to aid recall. This technique begins with a code to associate numbers with concrete items that the students can imagine or visualize. Sequencing and rhyming make recalling these associations easier. The associations become the pegs on which the items to be remembered are hung. Once learned, students can use the pegs to remember a variety of lists or sequences.

The following pegs can be taught to students within games. The peg words rhyme with the associated number, enhancing the connectiveness or association. Pages 291-292 provide a picture to go with each peg. You may reproduce these pictures for use in many different activities. The pegs for numbers one through nine are as follows:

Number	Peg Word
one	sun
two	shoe
three	bee
four	door
five	hive
six	ticks
seven	Kevin
eight	gate
nine	sign

Initial teaching of the pegs should be presented as a game, no matter the age of the student. Pacing is important, and the pace should be kept fairly rapid. Hold up the related picture as each word is mentioned. An example of a possible dialogue follows:

Teacher: Today we are going to play a game to help us remember pictures and relate them to a given number. Here's the first picture. (Display picture of *sun*.) It is number 1. For number 1, we will remember *sun*. Notice that "one" rhymes with "sun." Everybody, number 1 is . . .

Class: sun

Teacher: Number 2 is *shoe*. (Display picture of shoe.) Notice how the words rhyme. So every time I say number 2, you will get a picture in your mind of a (pause) *shoe*, and you will say . . .

Class: shoe

Teacher: Okay. (Display picture of sun.) When I say number one, you say . . .

Class: sun

Teacher: (Show picture of shoe.) When I say number 2, you say . . .

Class: shoe

Teacher: (Do not display a picture this time.) To review, 1 is . . .

Class: sun

Teacher: 2 is . . .

Class: shoe

Teacher: (Show picture of bee.) Number 3 is *bee*. Everybody get a picture in your mind of a bee. Your bee can look like the bee in this picture or you can think of your own bee. Does everybody have a picture of a bee? (pause) Number 3 is . . .

Class: bee

After introducing each new peg with its number, review all the previous peg and number connections. At the beginning, review sequentially. As students begin to connect the number with its visual image, the number peg associations should be reviewed in random order. Eventually, the pictures no longer need to be used. The pace of the lesson is important. It should be kept fairly fast to increase automaticity of visualizations, without being so fast that some students cannot keep up.

Some students will learn this system almost immediately, while others will need several review lessons. Younger students may benefit by initially using only four or five numbers. Once the majority of the students automatically make the associations, a variety of games can be played to encourage memorization of a series of unrelated objects.

Grocery list game

Students can be encouraged to use their peg numbers as a *magic* trick to amaze their parents and friends. Start by giving students a list of five grocery items to remember, associating each with a number and its peg. Increase to a series of nine items as students progress. An example dialogue to associate two items with the numbers one and two follows:

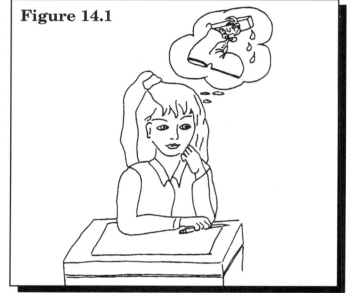

Figure 14.1

> Our first item on our grocery list is a carton of milk. Number 1 is the sun. Create a picture in your mind of the sun, then imagine the sun combined with milk in some way. Maybe the rays of the sun have become bottles of milk, or perhaps the sun is the shape of a large shining carton of milk. Do you have the picture? See the sun with its rays of milk bottles or whatever your picture is. (Pause to allow students to focus on their imagined association.) Okay, so number 1, sun, goes with . . .
>
> (Class: Milk.)
>
> Item two on our shopping list is butter. Number two is . . .
>
> (Class: Shoe.)
>
> Can you imagine the butter inside a shoe? It might be a tub of butter in the shoe or maybe the shoe is stepping on a stick of butter, whatever works for you. Can you see it, picture it, visualize it? (Pause) Now let's review . . .

The First Nine Presidents

The peg system can serve as a cue to help students remember the names of the first nine presidents. A caution, however, is that this system only serves as a cue to remember something already known. It will not work if the students do not know the names of the Presidents; the pegs are a trigger to recall items in a given order. After the students discuss the nine Presidents, peg words can be used as associations to help remember their names in order. The following exemplifies teaching the associations for the first five Presidents. It is most helpful for students to develop their own images, although some students need more guidance and examples than others. If the group can handle it, encourage multiple responses for the visualizations, as this strengthens individuality in the response patterns.

Teacher:	Class, remember the peg words we learned before? Let's review. (Allow time for the class to respond using each peg word: 1 is sun, 2 is shoe, 3 is bee, 4 is door, 5 is hive, 6 is ticks, 7 is Kevin, 8 is gate, 9 is sign.)
	Remember our unit on the first nine Presidents of the United States? We are now going to use our peg words to help us remember the order of the first nine Presidents.
	Okay, President 1 is Washington. What is our word for 1? Right, it's sun. Can you picture some *washing* hanging out in the sun? The wash is on a clothesline and it is hanging in the bright sun. See it. Feel the hot sun. (Pause briefly to allow students to focus on their image.) Remember: one—sun—washing. Our first President is . . .
Class:	Washington
Teacher:	Good. President 2 is Adams. Our word for 2 is (pause) shoe. What can you imagine to connect shoe and Adams?
Student:	A shoe hitting someone's *Adam's apple.*
Teacher:	Good. Can you see it? Picture the shoe coming right toward your Adam's apple. See it. Touch your Adam's apple. (Pause) Remember: two—shoe—Adam's apple. So we remember President 2 is . . .
Class:	Adams
	(Review the two associations. Use cues such as "see it," "picture it," and "feel it" to encourage students to visualize the associations.)
Teacher:	President 3 is Jefferson. Our word for 3 is (pause) bee. What do you see (visualize) here?
Student:	*Jeff's son* is running away from a bunch of bees that are flying toward him.
Teacher:	Good. Hear the bees. See the bees. See *Jeff's son* wrapping himself in *fur.* Can you see Jeff's son wrapped in the fur? What does it remind us of? Jefferson. See it. Hear the bees. See the bees going toward Jeff's son wrapped in fur. Picture it. (Pause)

	Remember: three—bee—Jeff's son in fur. So we remember President 3 is . . .
Class:	Jefferson.
	(Review the three associations. Encourage the students to visualize and picture the images. Then review the three presidents in random order as quickly as possible without leaving any students behind.)
Teacher:	President 4 is Madison. What's our word for 4? (door) What do you see here?
Student:	I see a man who is *mad at his son* so he is slamming the door.
Teacher:	Excellent. Imagine him slamming a door real hard. See the door slam. Hear the door slam. Why is he slamming the door?
Class:	Because he is mad at his son!
Teacher:	Right, 4 is Madison. Our word is door, so we think of a man who is mad at his son so he slams the door. Picture it. See it. Hear it. Feel the vibration of the door slamming. Remember: four—door—mad at his son. (Pause) So we remember President 4 is . . .
Class:	Madison
	(Review the four associations. Review them in sequence, forward, and backward, then in random order.)
Teacher:	President 5 is Monroe. Our word for 5 is hive.
Student:	Can we use the movie star, Marilyn Monroe? We can picture Marilyn *Monroe* with a giant beehive hairdo (demonstrating a very large hairdo).
Teacher:	Good. Can everyone see it? Picture it. See Marilyn Monroe with that huge beehive hairdo. (Pause) Remember: five—hive—Monroe with hive hairdo. So we remember President 5 is . . .
Class:	Monroe.

Remember to review after you establish each new association. Following are suggestions for associations for the next four presidents. You and your students may develop others.

- President J. Q. Adams—6 is ticks; picture a curly **J** and a curly **Q** wiggling with the ticks. Students may use their pinky finger to draw a curly **J** in the air to add some movement.

The Source for Dyslexia & Dysgraphia
Copyright © 1999 LinguiSystems, Inc.

- President Jackson—7 is Kevin; picture a boy with Kevin written on his shirt playing jacks.

- President Van Buren—8 is gate; picture a van burning by a big gate.

- President Harrison—9 is a sign; picture a hairy son holding a sign, such as a picket sign.

Multiplication tables

The pegs can be used to help teach and reinforce the multiplication facts. For many dyslexics, the rote recall necessary for remembering these facts causes substantial difficulty and this system, which combines imagery and mnemonics, can help them bypass their struggles with rote sequential recall. The system, called MFM: Memory Foundations for Multiplication, can supplement any general classroom approach and is useful in several different situations:

- When first presenting multiplication facts

- As remediation for students who have struggled with traditional techniques

- As a creative approach to learning and reviewing facts for all students

Some children will find the MFM system more cumbersome than merely memorizing the facts. This is well and good because if rote memorization is that easy, these students do not need an alternate system. However, children who struggle with memorization of rote information gain an important connective link using MFM.

Prerequisites to MFM

Students need to understand several concepts before beginning to understand multiplication. These prerequisites are especially critical for dyslexics to increase their understanding of the process. These concepts are:

- Place value

- Addition is increasing the value of the number (the number becomes larger)

- Subtraction is decreasing the value of the number (the number becomes smaller)

- Multiplication is a form of addition (3 + 3 + 3 is the same as 3 three times, or 3 x 3)

To be successful with multiplication, students also need to master several skills, such as the following:

- The ability to sequence random numbers, at least up through five digits

- The ability to set up and represent an addition problem using manipulatives

- The ability to set up and represent an addition problem using numbers

- The ability to set up and represent a subtraction problem using manipulatives, placing the larger number on top

- The ability to set up and represent a subtraction problem using numbers

- The ability to set up and represent a multiplication problem using manipulatives, indicating understanding that multiplication is the repeated adding of equal groups

- The ability to reverse the multiplier order of a problem (2 x 3 and 3 x 2) and understand why the answer remains the same

The MFM System

As students learn the MFM system, they must be persuaded that learning the multiplication facts is not an overwhelming task. Although 100 basic multiplication facts are involved in learning the tables for 1 through 10 (shown in Figure 14.2), not all 100 facts need to be memorized. The 100 facts can be reduced to only 21 facts by eliminating those that are easily learned and combinations that are reversible. This enhances the connectiveness of the learning. Eliminations can be demonstrated by the following example, either on an overhead projector or on the chalkboard. First, display a typical 10 x 10 multiplication chart.

Figure 14.2

X	1	2	3	4	5	6	7	8	9	10
1	1	2	3	4	5	6	7	8	9	10
2	2	4	6	8	10	12	14	16	18	20
3	3	6	9	12	15	18	21	24	27	30
4	4	8	12	16	20	24	28	32	36	40
5	5	10	15	20	25	30	35	40	45	50
6	6	12	18	24	30	36	42	48	54	60
7	7	14	21	28	35	42	49	56	63	70
8	8	16	24	32	40	48	56	64	72	80
9	9	18	27	36	45	54	63	72	81	90
10	10	20	30	40	50	60	70	80	90	100

It is easy to see that there are 100 multiplication facts. The first question to ask the students is, "Do we need to memorize the 1's facts?" The children should, through discovery, realize that there is no need to memorize the 1's facts because the product of any number and 1 is that number. Once they realize this, the "1" row and the "1" column can be erased, as in the chart in Figure 14.3 on page 271.

Now there are only 81 facts remaining to be learned. The next question is, "Do we need to memorize the 2's facts?" Lead students to discover the answer.

Figure 14.3—1's eliminated

X	1	2	3	4	5	6	7	8	9	10
1										
2		4	6	8	10	12	14	16	18	20
3		6	9	12	15	18	21	24	27	30
4		8	12	16	20	24	28	32	36	40
5		10	15	20	25	30	35	40	45	50
6		12	18	24	30	36	42	48	54	60
7		14	21	28	35	42	49	56	63	70
8		16	24	32	40	48	56	64	72	80
9		18	27	36	45	54	63	72	81	90
10		20	30	40	50	60	70	80	90	100

Figure 14.4—2's eliminated

X	1	2	3	4	5	6	7	8	9	10
1										
2										
3			9	12	15	18	21	24	27	30
4			12	16	20	24	28	32	36	40
5			15	20	25	30	35	40	45	50
6			18	24	30	36	42	48	54	60
7			21	28	35	42	49	56	63	70
8			24	32	40	48	56	64	72	80
9			27	36	45	54	63	72	81	90
10			30	40	50	60	70	80	90	100

Figure 14.5—5's eliminated

X	1	2	3	4	5	6	7	8	9	10
1										
2										
3			9	12			18	21	24	27	30
4			12	16			24	28	32	36	40
5										
6			18	24			36	42	48	54	60
7			21	28			42	49	56	63	70
8			24	32			48	56	64	72	80
9			27	36			54	63	72	81	90
10			30	40			60	70	80	90	100

These do not need to be memorized because we can count by 2's to find the answer. For example, 3 x 2 is the same as counting by 2's three times (2, 4, 6). Also, any number times 2 is the same as adding that number to itself. For example, 6 x 2 is the same as 6 + 6. It is critical that each student understands these basic concepts of multiplication.

Once the students realize they do not need to memorize the 2's tables, the "2" column and the "2" row can be erased, as has been done in the chart in Figure 14.4. Sixty-four facts remain to be learned. The next question is, "Do we need to memorize the 5's tables?" Most students know how to count by 5's, which is reinforced by telling time and counting nickels. Students should be able to conclude that counting by 5's will give them the answer to any of the 5's facts. For example, to discover the answer for 6 x 5, students need only to count by 5 six times: 5, 10, 15, 20, 25, 30. At this point, the "5" row and the "5" column can be erased because these facts do not have to be memorized, as in the chart in Figure 14.5.

Only 49 facts remain. The next question to ask is, "Do we have to memorize the 10's facts?" Many tricks are easily used to determine the product of any number times 10, especially single-digit numbers. One trick is counting by 10's. Another way is to place a zero after the number. Once students understand these concepts, the "10" row and the "10" column can be erased from the chart, as in Figure 14.6.

There are now only 36 facts remaining in the chart. The next question is, "Are there any duplicate combinations that we can eliminate? If we memorize 4 x 6 = 24, do we also have to memorize 6 x 4 = 24?" The obvious answer is "no," and it is vital that students understand the concept of reversibility before proceeding. At that point, the duplication combinations can be erased, as in the chart in Figure 14.7.

Students now have only 21 facts remaining. The MFM system deals with these 21 facts.

Using the MFM System

Step 1: **Review peg words.** Review the picture clues for numbers 1 through 9 using the peg system. Correct any errors immediately so each student's connections become automatic and efficient. Use a variety of the following techniques to review the pictures and to help students generalize their learning.

- Repeat each number and picture in unison with the class.

- Match each picture to its number and then match each number to its picture, progressing in sequence.

- Match a picture to a number or a number to a picture, progressing in random order.

- Use auditory input (name) and verbal response (for example, you say "bee" and the class says "3").

- Use visual input with verbal response (for example, you show

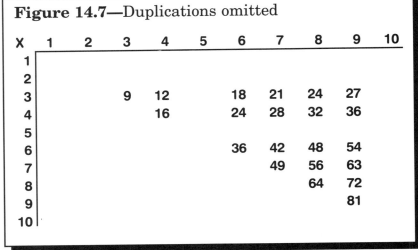

Figure 14.6—10's eliminated

X	1	2	3	4	5	6	7	8	9	10
1										
2										
3			9	12		18	21	24	27	
4			12	16		24	28	32	36	
5										
6			18	24		36	42	48	54	
7			21	28		42	49	56	63	
8			24	32		48	56	64	72	
9			27	36		54	63	72	81	
10										

Figure 14.7—Duplications omitted

X	1	2	3	4	5	6	7	8	9	10
1										
2										
3			9	12		18	21	24	27	
4				16		24	28	32	36	
5										
6						36	42	48	54	
7							49	56	63	
8								64	72	
9									81	
10										

The Source for Dyslexia & Dysgraphia
Copyright © 1999 LinguiSystems, Inc.

Figure 14.8—Bee times bee equals sign.

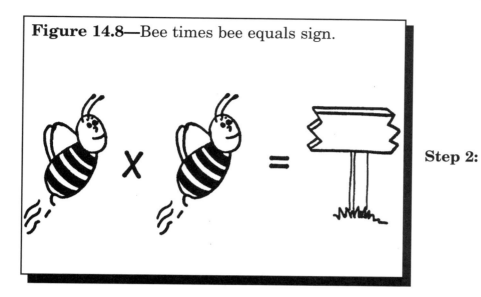

Figure 14.9—Bee times door equals a sun and a shoe.

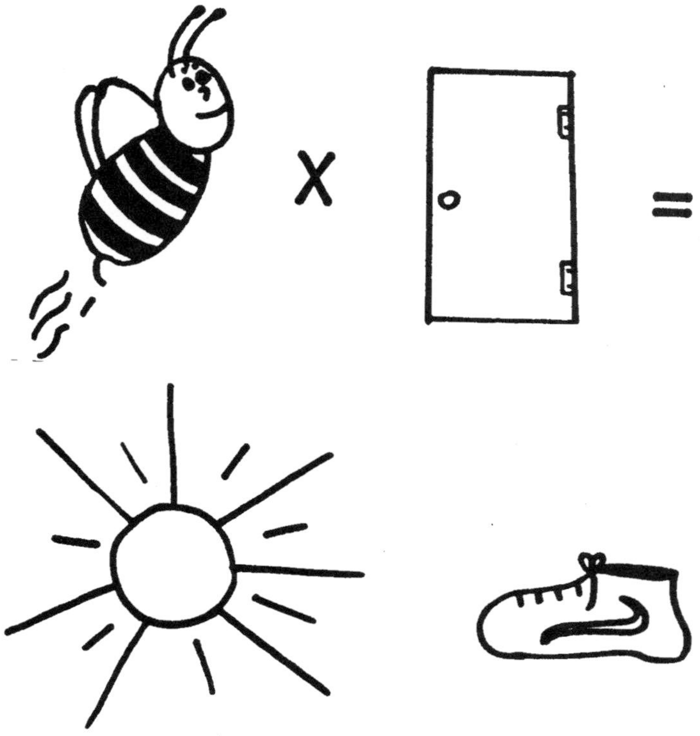

the number 3 and the class says "bee").

- Use a combination of auditory and visual input with verbal response.

Step 2: **Establish links.** Use MFM pictures and poems. (The 21 MFM pictures and accompanying poems are found on pages 293-298.) Create the picture for 3 x 3 using two bees and a sign. Ask, "What do you see?" (two bees and a sign) Put in a multiplication sign (x) and an equal sign (=), as in Figure 14.8. Say, "Let's change this picture to numbers using our pegs. What would that be?" After the students respond, write 3 x 3 = 9 underneath the related pictures. Read the corresponding poem with the students and then ask, "How does this poem help us?" Encourage a discussion about the relationship of the poem to the multiplication fact. To help reinforce the poem, give students a copy of the poem and have them draw the pictures of the two bees and a sign.

Step 3: **Use the pictures.** Make copies of each peg word picture. This step is best performed using one set at the front of the room as a demonstration for the class while providing two sets to each pair of students.

The following steps may be combined in a single lesson, especially with older students. For younger students, focus on only one step per lesson, combining steps as part of the review process.

1. Read a given poem. (For example, *The bee by the door has a good view;/ He sees the sun wearing a shoe./ Three times four is a one and a two.*) Have students set up the picture sequence by selecting the appropriate pictures and placing them in the correct order as the poem is read, as in Figures 14.9, but without the x and = signs. The students add the x and = signs after the pictures are set up.

2. The teacher sets up the pictures on a clear board while the students say the poem. Then have them *read* the pictures: "Bee times door is 3 x 4. That equals sun and shoe or a one and a two—that's twelve."

3. Students say the poem while again arranging their own pictures into the correct sequence. They then *read* the pictures again.

4. Students say the poem and then use manipulatives (such as blocks) to represent the numbers, for example, four groups of three. This is an important step to reinforce the connections.

Step 4: **Review.** Review the poems, pictures, and math facts using the sequence in Step 3 (using the pictures) or one of the following alternatives:

- MFM flash cards. Show the picture representing 3 x 3; students say aloud "equals 9."

- MFM flash cards with poem. Show a fact such as 3 x 3; students say the poem.

- Periodic timed tests, including all facts taught up to that point. When students perform the timed test, encourage them to use the strategy rather than using their fingers. For example, you might say, "I'm timing you, but don't rush. When you get stuck, stop, look at the numbers, and try to remember the strategy. You can quietly say the poem." It is best to postpone using the timed tests until students are fairly solid on all of the 3's facts.

When students first take the timed tests, place all the facts in order. As students advance, begin to rearrange the order of the facts. As students gain proficiency in the facts they have learned, add other facts, such as the 1's facts, the 2's facts or the 5's. Have students take each timed test several times. Their initial time establishes a baseline. Each time they retake a test, their goal is to improve their own scores. They should chart how many facts they are able to get correct within one minute to provide a visual representation of their progress. This motivates and generates confidence in their new skills. Their only competition should be to improve their own time.

Additional suggestions for MFM
- Use manipulatives such as Cuisenaire rods, link blocks, or counters to reinforce the concept that multiplication is an array of facts. As an example, an array for 6 x 3 would be:

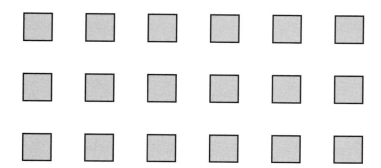

- Discourage finger counting; encourage the use of the strategy.

- Present no more than two or three facts per session to ensure that students are confident with each connection and poem. For this strategy to be successful, it is important for students to use the poem or picture connection to come up with the facts within a few seconds.

- Use constant review, spiraling through various procedures and steps. Start each session with a review of all facts taught in previous sessions.

- When using the poems, some teachers prefer to omit the tens because they have not taught base 10. Although it is more accurate to use the tens ("3 x 4 is 1 ten and 2"), some prefer to leave it out and just say, "3 x 4 is a 1 and a 2." If your students have been taught base 10, it is more accurate to use the tens. To do so, change the answer in each poem to include them. For example:

  Three times four is one **ten** and a two.
  Three times six is one **ten** and an eight.
  Three times seven is two **tens** and a one.
  Three times eight is two **tens** and a four.

Mnemonics

Mnemonics refer to memory links, or memory cues. It is a Greek word meaning "pertaining to memory." The word comes from *Mnemosyne* (/ne-mo'-sin-ne/), the Greek goddess of memory and the mother of Muses. Mnemonics can stimulate spatial, visual, and rhythmic strengths, enabling students to better remember details or rote sequential information. Just as many children learn commercials and jingles rapidly, they will also learn silly mnemonic sentences and remember them longer. Mnemonics use a pattern to create the memory link.

Caution:	Complex mnemonics do not always work with language-impaired students. For these students, mnemonics need to be very concrete.

Previously in this book, the mnemonic COPS was discussed as a system to help students remember to proof their work in four separate steps. The MFR and MFM systems presented visual mnemonics to help students retain and recall sound/symbol correspondences and multiplication facts. Following are two more examples using mnemonics. The first uses kinesthetic mnemonics to help with the 9's times tables. The second creates the mnemonic links to remember the tricky parts of spelling words.

Caution:	Too many mnemonics taught at any one time can create confusion rather than clarity.

Prerequisites for teaching finger mnemonics for the 9's tables

There are patterns within many of the multiplication tables, but often students do not automatically become aware of such number patterns. Consequently, patterns should be explicitly taught. The 9's table, for example, presents a very interesting pattern. To help students become aware of the pattern, write the 9's table on the chalkboard in a vertical column, as follows, making sure the ones column in the products (answers) are lined up:

9 x 1 =   9
9 x 2 = 18
9 x 3 = 27
9 x 4 = 36
9 x 5 = 45
9 x 6 = 54
9 x 7 = 63
9 x 8 = 72
9 x 9 = 81
9 x 10 = 90

Figure 14.10

X	1	2	3	4	5	6	7	8	9	10
1	1	2	3	4	5	6	7	8	9	10
2	2	4	6	8	10	12	14	16	18	20
3	3	6	9	12	15	18	21	24	27	30
4	4	8	12	16	20	24	28	32	36	40
5	5	10	15	20	25	30	35	40	45	50
6	6	12	18	24	30	36	42	48	54	60
7	7	14	21	28	35	42	49	56	63	70
8	8	16	24	32	40	48	56	64	72	80
9	9	18	27	36	45	54	63	72	81	90
10	10	20	30	40	50	60	70	80	90	100

Point to the column with the products and have the students look at the digits in the ones place and identify any relationship among the numbers that they may see. Then have them look at the digits in the tens place and describe any number pattern they may see. Lead them to notice that the digits in the ones place progress in descending order and the digits in the tens place progress in ascending order.

There are some other number patterns involving 9's. It is easy to think of 10 more and then minus one. For example, assume a student knows this equation:

9 x 3 is 27 (or 9 + 9 + 9 = 27)

Then 9 x 4 can be computed by thinking the following:

27 + 9 = 27 + 10 (37) - 1 (36)

This pattern also becomes very evident to students if they look at a multiplication grid, as in Figure 14.10. They might also notice that the digits in each answer add up to nine and that the last five answers are the same as the first five answers, only reversed.

Students who enjoy tactile cues, and students who need to move to learn (and are often wiggly in a classroom) may find finger multiplication an efficient strategy. Students generally use their fingers only as long as doing so is necessary. Once they master the facts, they naturally eliminate the crutches, except perhaps to check on specific difficult facts. Some students rely on using their fingers longer than others. For these students, using their fingers may provide their primary access to learning specific facts.

Finger 9's, One Digit

The finger system for the 9's table is relatively easy. Students begin by placing both hands in front of them, on a table, palm side down with fingers outstretched. The students mentally number each finger starting with the pinky on the left hand (as in Figure 14.11). (Note: All the illustrations of these steps appear on pages 279-281.) Younger students or students who have difficulty visualizing can be helped by placing a numbered circle or small sticker on the corresponding finger.

1. This finger system for 9's works when multiplying 9 by a single digit. For example, to multiply 9 by 5, students fold in their number five finger, as in Figure 14.12.

2. Students then count the fingers to the left of their folded finger and the total becomes the 10's digit. The number of fingers to the right of the folded finger becomes the 1's digit. Students then have the answer. In this case, it is four 10's (to the left) and five 1's (to the right), or 45, as in Figure 14.13.

3. Have students practice with 9 x 7. The seventh finger is put down and then the number of 10's is counted (six) and the number of 1's (three). The answer is 63, as in Figure 14.14.

4. Practice this procedure with all single-digit 9 facts and students will notice how easy it becomes. It also works with 9 x 10, as indicated in Figure 14.15.

Finger 9's, 2 digits

The procedure for 1-digit problems can be modified and used to multiply 9 by any 2-digit number, as long as the first digit is smaller than the second. Students place their hands flat on the table, palm side down with the fingers outstretched. Again, each finger is numbered starting with the pinky on the left.

1. To multiply 9 x 36, students first multiply the ones digit (the 6) using the same method just described, as shown in Figure 14.16. The 5 fingers to the left of the bent finger represent the 10's, and the 4 fingers to the right of the bent finger represent the 1's, representing 9 x 6 = 54.

2. Now the 3 in 36 needs to be manipulated. From the left, count three fingers (to represent the 3 in 36). Separate these fingers from the group using a pencil or stick, as in Figure 14.17.

3. Now there are 3 groups of fingers: a group of 3, a group of 2, and a group of 4. These groups represent the number 324, which is the product of 9 x 36.

4. As another example, multiply 9 x 57. First bend the 7 finger, leaving 6 fingers on the left and 3 on the right, as in Figure 14.18.

5. Then separate 5 fingers on the left to form a group. This results in 3 groups of fingers: 5, 1, and 3, as in Figure 14.19. The answer to 9 x 57 is 513.

Caution:	The first digit in the number to be multiplied must be smaller than the second for the 9's times two digits to work.

Figure 14.11—Numbering of fingers for 9s.

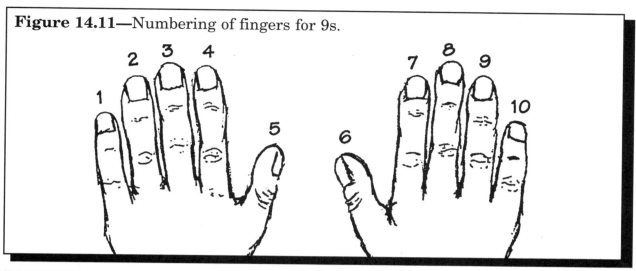

Figure 14.12—Process for figuring 9 x 5.

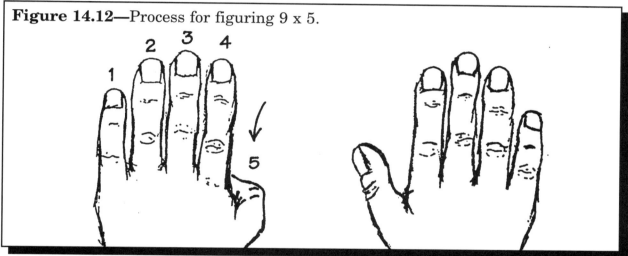

Figure 14.13—Answer to 9 x 5.

Step 1: Count tens, 4 tens.   Step 2: Count ones, 5 ones.

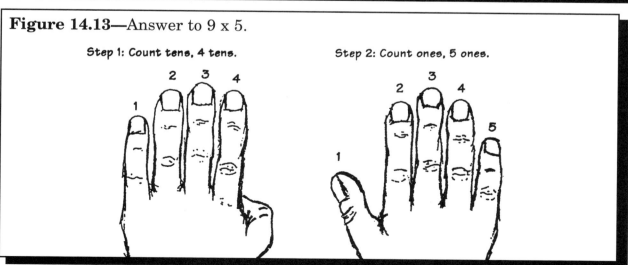

Figure 14.14—Process for figuring 9 x 7.

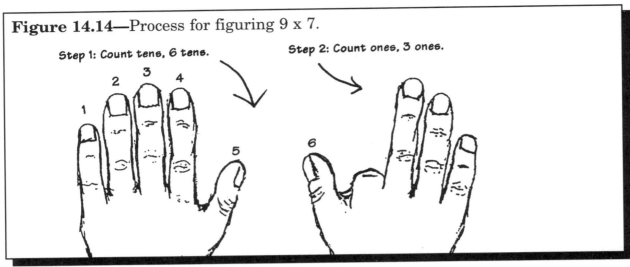

Figure 14.15—Process for figuring 9 x 10.

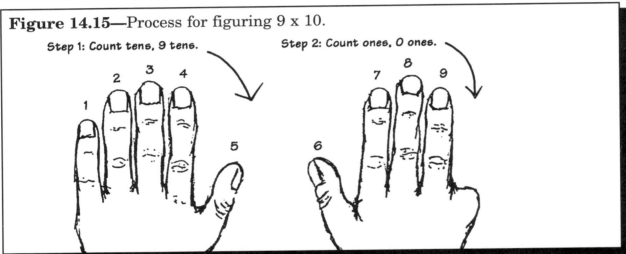

Figure 14.16—The first step, 9 x 6, in figuring 9 x 36.

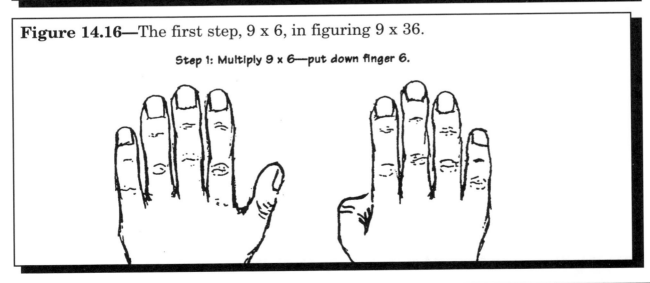

The Source for Dyslexia & Dysgraphia
Copyright © 1999 LinguiSystems, Inc.

Figure 14.17—The second and third steps in figuring 9 x 36. 9 x 36 = 324.

Step 2: Separate 3 from the group, starting at left.
Step 3: Write down the numbers: 3 hundreds, 2 tens, 4 ones. 9 x 36 = 324.

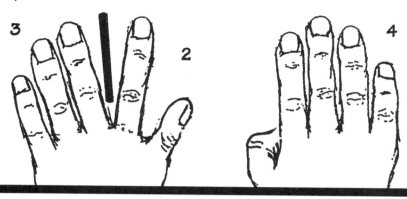

Figure 14.18—The first step, 9 x 7, in figuring 9 x 57.

Step 1: Multiply 9 x 7—put down finger 7.

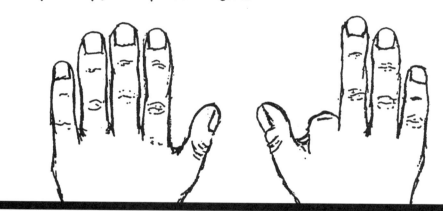

Figure 14.19—The second and third steps in figuring 9 x 57. 9 x 57 = 513.

Step 2: Separate 5 from the group.
Step 3: Write down the numbers: 5 hundreds, 1 ten, 3 ones. 9 x 57 = 513.

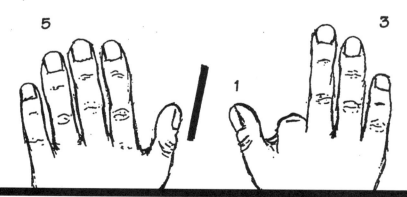

Figure 14.20

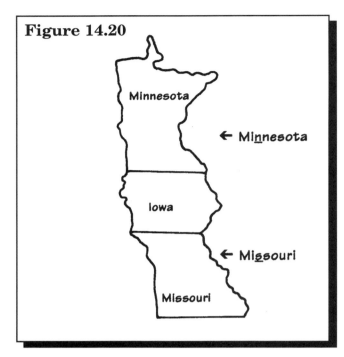

As a review, the students can be presented with a pattern (using your actual hands or pictures of hands on a board or overhead). Students then determine and write down the problem and the answer that is represented. This activity will increase their ability to *read* their fingers and visualize the 9's facts.

Use of mnemonics with content areas

Creating mnemonics can be quite fun and lead to noticing many innovative associations. For example, in geography, students might be learning locations of the 50 states. Many times, dyslexic students confuse similar words such as *Minnesota* and *Missouri*. If a student is trying to learn Iowa's borders, she may notice a helpful mnemonic cue. Mi**nn**esota is north of Iowa and has two n's. Mi**ss**ouri is south of Iowa and has two s's. Refer to Figure 14.20.

Basic mnemonics for spelling

Dyslexic students always have varying degrees of difficulty with spelling. An important aspect of learning spelling (besides phonological awareness and phonetic analysis) is to have a system for remembering the tricky parts of spelling words, is presented in Chapter 11. A system, especially a mnemonic system, enhances the eidetics, or automatic visual recognition. Remember, students can become overwhelmed with too many mnemonics at one time.

Using the five spelling mnemonic strategies in Chapter 11, try to create your own mnemonics to help you remember how to spell the following words. Create your own cues before looking at the suggestions below.

- friend
- attorney
- prey
- knowledge
- comedy
- announce
- canoe
- reign
- recruit
- tragedy
- recognize

Caution: Don't look at the next page until you have developed your own cues.

Suggestions:

- *Friend:* Look for another word in friend. Then create a related sentence (strategy 2 or 3). *end*
  A fri**end** to the **end**. or **I** am with my fr**i**end.

- *Canoe:* The tricky part is **oe**. Think of a common word that ends in **oe** with the same sound (strategy 2). *shoe*
  This can**oe** looks like my sh**oe**.

- *Attorney:* There are two tricky parts here: **orn** and **ey**. Think of words containing those segments and create a sentence (strategy 2). *key, torn*
  The **key** has **torn** the attorney's shirt.

- *Reign:* Since the whole sequence of letters is tricky, an acronym will work well. Include the word *rulers* to associate the meaning (strategy 4).
  Rulers **e**at **i**cy **g**rapes **n**ow.

- *Prey:* The tricky part is **ey**. Think of a rhyming word that ends in **ey** (strategy 2). *they*
  Th**ey** like the pr**ey**.

- *Recruit:* The difficult part is **uit**. Make a sentence using a rhyming word (strategy 2). *suit*
  The recr**uit** has a new **suit**.

- *Knowledge*: Relate to the root of *know* (strategy 5).
  Knowledge, as we **know**, is very important.

- *Tragedy:* Look for another word within (strategy 2). age
  the **age** of trag**e**dy

- *Comedy:* The tricky part is the middle **e**. Look for another word within comedy (strategy 2). *come*
  Come to the com**e**dy.

- *Recognize:* This word works well with a mispronunciation (strategy 1).
  re-cog-nize

- *Announce:* Look for other words within (strategy 2). *Ann, ounce*
  Ann weighs an **ounce**.

Mind Maps

Mind maps (also known as visual organizers) provide a technique for organizing information. Because such organizers are open-ended, they increase the rapid connection of the thought patterns and provide immediate feedback. Visual organizers were discussed as important for pre-organizing ideas for written expression. They can also be used as a study skill technique to increase active reading and provide a valuable aid to recall.

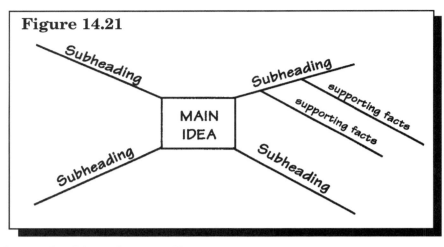

Figure 14.21

Mind mapping before reading a chapter

Students can place the main idea in the center of a page and each subheading from a chapter (usually printed in the book as a dark section subtitle) on a line coming out of the main idea. This will help preview the story or chapter. As they read each section, they can write key words for the supporting facts under the appropriate subheading, as in Figure 14.21. This pattern allows students to insert information as they encounter it and place it where they feel it is important, knowing they can rearrange it at any time.

Mind mapping to increase active reading

It is very important to help students become more active in their reading process rather than just moving their eyes across the lines of print. One technique is to encourage the use of two colors of Post-it® notes. As the student reads a section, one color Post-it® can be used to summarize the main idea. The second color Post-it® can be used to write key words or phrases for the facts that support the main idea. After finishing the chapter, students can reorganize their notes into a mind map or other visual organizer, selecting from the variety of formats on pages 253-256.

Strategies for using mind mapping

Following are some basic suggestions that are helpful when students create mind maps or visual organizers.

- Use unlined paper.
- Print or write neatly.
- Use color to differentiate categories.
- Use connecting lines.
- Use a variety of images and symbols.

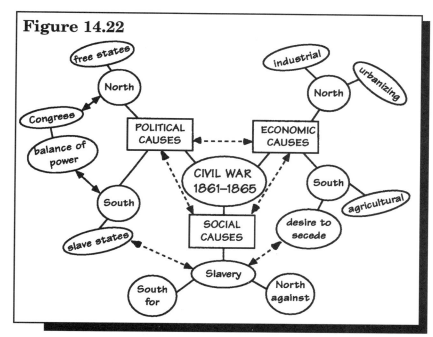

Figure 14.22

- Use arrows, codes, and symbols to show connections and associations among different groups.
- Draw boxes or rings around groups of concepts and images to create units.

Figure 14.22 represents a more complex mind map of the Civil War, reprinted from *Your Child's Growing Mind*, by Jane Healy, ©1987, used by permission of Doubleday, a division of Bantam Doubleday Dell Publishing Group, Inc.

Metaphors

Metaphors and other associative techniques provide a link between a familiar concept and new information. It is one of the most powerful ways to link characteristics and enhance recall. The learner's goal is to create and then enhance the link between the familiar and the unfamiliar by linking some common traits. Metaphors create a synthesis between more global visual strategies that can be imaged and more detailed verbal labels and/or characteristics. Example questions that encourage this associative technique are:

- What do you know that is like ____?
- How are they alike? How are they different?
- What _____ is like this? (animal/machine/color/cloth)

These questions can be extended to, "What do you do when you're cold? How is that like mercury?"

Metaphors are frequently used in the teaching process to help students understand new ideas by explaining these ideas in terms of something the students already understand. For example, "Global learning is like seeing the whole view, similar to how an eagle flying sees the large view of the land below," or "The three branches of government are related to each other, just like the three parts of my bike." Helping students create their own metaphors emphasizes these valuable connections. Students who are skilled at making connections as part of their learning process benefit dramatically from the use of metaphors and find that they are more successful in test-taking situations because their knowledge goes beyond the rote and has more depth.

Students with language-based learning disabilities such as dyslexia often have difficulty asking questions to clarify what they do not understand. When they state, "I don't understand," it does not tell a teacher what aspect of the concept needs to be clarified. However, if the student asks a question using a metaphor, such as "Is a kidney like a coffee filter in how it works?" the teacher can explain the similarities and differences between the two items. This is an important skill for students to develop, especially for use in general education classes.

Young students can be encouraged to think of using metaphors by asking them to make comparisons. They can complete sentences such as:

- Dogs smell like ____.
- School is like ____.
- Water feels like ____.

They can also play a game similar to I Spy. Instead of saying, "I spy something blue," the children can use phrases such as, "I spy something that is like a soft crayon" (*chalk*) or "I spy something that is like a hook to keep papers together." (*staple*).

Another activity to begin the use of metaphors, especially with young students can be to show students pictures of two objects and ask them to describe the similarities. Encourage them to consider color, material, texture, size, shape, and function. Some examples include:

- A sofa and a chair (you sit on both)
- A pencil and a crayon (both are used for writing on paper)
- A head and a ball (both are round)
- The sky and a blue flower (both are blue)

As a variation, students can cut out several pictures of items from magazines. They can paste the pictures in a vertical line on large pieces of paper. They go through the magazines again to find pictures of objects that have a characteristic that is similar to each item in their list. For example, if their initial list includes scissors, they may add a picture of a knife because both are used for cutting.

Using metaphors with older students

Metaphors can be used to stimulate students' thinking about new concepts in content areas. For example, to define *infinity*, they could say, "It's like looking in a mirror and seeing yourself see yourself." Consider the difference between two groups of students studying the concept of infinity of space. In one situation, the students look up definitions in dictionaries and find a few examples in a textbook of facts such as the size of the universe and the duration of time.

Figure 14.23

The 13 Colonies Rap

Let's take a little trip to the northern colonies,
Where fish and ships and wood will be.
Massachusetts is found here,
The Mayflower landed very near.
Rhode Island is found right below,
It's so small, where'd it go?
Right next to it is Connecticut,
Look to the left and you'll find it.
Way up north is New Hampshire,
It's pretty cold, so bring your fur.

New York, New Jersey, middle colonies,
Lots of bread and a lot of Yankees.
Pennsylvania or William Penn's woods,
Land of Quakers and Brotherhood.
Delaware, Delaware, small colony,
Was the first state that came to be.

I don't know, but from word of mouth,
The place to be is in the South.
In the Carolinas, South and North,
Where peas and corn and rice came forth.
The first colony was Virginia,
It was the start of America.
There was a place called Maryland,
It gave its people free religion.
Georgia is a land with peach,
This song is fun, what a way to teach.

These students memorize and give information back. In the other situation, the teacher brings in two mirrors and initiates a discussion of the metaphor as a means of explaining and exploring the concept of immeasurability. The teacher asks the students to generate metaphors of their own, related to the concept.

The second method is considerably more interesting to students. It provides for dynamic engagement and produces a deeper, clearer understanding of the concept of infinity as something that goes on and on. This type of hands-on, connective learning is especially valuable for dyslexic students.

Other ways to stimulate students' thinking is to have them compare something they know with a new concept that is being introduced. An example is, "How is a revolution like a volcano?" or "How are kidneys like a coffee filter?" Students can brainstorm characteristics of each item, writing all of the characteristics for one item in one list, then for the other item in another list. The two lists can be compared to identify similarities and differences. If desired, a Venn diagram can be created. (See the Visual Organizer on page 255.)

Older students can also be encouraged to search for examples of metaphoric language in TV commercials and magazine ads. Examples of questions to stimulate students' thinking include:

- Which word in this ad has two meanings?
- What is the meaning you expect when you first see the word?
- What is the second meaning?
- How are these two meanings (or ideas) alike?
- How are they different?

Music and Rhythm

Music, rhythm, and movement are effective techniques that help create a relaxed learning atmosphere. They enhance integration of processing strategies and help students create links, especially among linear rote sequential information. Examples include strengthening reading skills through choral reading or the chanting of spelling words. Singing multiplication tables has been helpful for many students. Chanting or remembering science or social studies information is also quite valuable. An example of a rap created for a group of dyslexic students to help review their unit on the original 13 colonies is included in Figure 14.23. This rap was used after the students had already studied a map, knew the 13 names, and understood the concept of the colonies and the importance of their establishment.

Creativity and imagination are the most important aspects for developing activities that include music and rhythm to enhance students' success. Many times, once these strategies are modeled, students begin to create their own raps or songs. This is when the most powerful recall strategies are created.

Teaching Strategies That Benefit Dyslexic Learners

Strategy	Specific tasks
Multisensory presentations	• Present information using a variety of sensory inputs ✔ for skill development ✔ for concept explanations • Encourage hands-on learning & manipulations • Help student build pathways using a variety of sensory modalities • Provide interactive involvement with the ideas, concepts
Connective learning and dynamic engagement with materials	• Make connections among and between learning tasks and real world experience • Apply ideas to daily life and/or familiar situations • Build on what students already know • Make links between an activity and the concepts to be learned • Engage students with the materials & ideas • Provide new learning within context of familiar experiences
Metacognitive awareness *definition*: awareness of strategies needed to perform a task as well as ability to employ self-regulation skills such as planning, evaluating, monitoring, and modifying	• Use metacognitive skills in: ✔ Writing ✔ Reading & spelling ✔ Math ✔ Content areas • Use to help student organize and plan • Encourage self-questioning techniques • Ensure that students understand reasons for task
Spiraling	• Review and repeat previously presented material • Connect past learning to present material • Provide variety: not all students relate in the same way to every activity; variety enhances the chances for multiple pathways in the brain to categorize information
Imagery	• Visual images enhance dynamic engagement • Back up verbal explanations with visual charts, graphs, pictures, demonstrations • Use words to help students create images • Images can be visual, kinesthetic, auditory, or tactile
Mnemonic strategies	• Can be visual, verbal and/or motor mnemonics • Use as strategies for: ✔ Rote recall of facts or procedures ✔ Organization ✔ Higher order thinking skills ✔ Visual organization strategies

continued on the next page

Teaching Strategies That Benefit Dyslexic Learners

Strategy	Specific tasks
Mind mapping	• Use visual pictures/designs • Preview material to be covered • Provides a global, whole picture overview • Allows for nonlinear, associative connections
Metaphors, analogies, & associations	• Provides connections & lateral learning to increase depth and breadth of learning • Use real life stories & associations • Plan a variety of activities around any learning to make stronger associations and connections • Use to connect something new to something familiar
Music and rhythm	• Associates new information in a dynamic manner • Provides another recall pathway to hook in information • Increases spiraling of information • Encourages students to develop another framework for the information • The rhythm and tune connects concepts and facts
Positive statements (Dyslexics often have fragile self-concepts.)	• Place positive affirmations on the wall and use for discussion; change frequently • Create a positive emotional environment for learning • Phrase statements positively: "remember your homework" rather than "don't forget . . ."

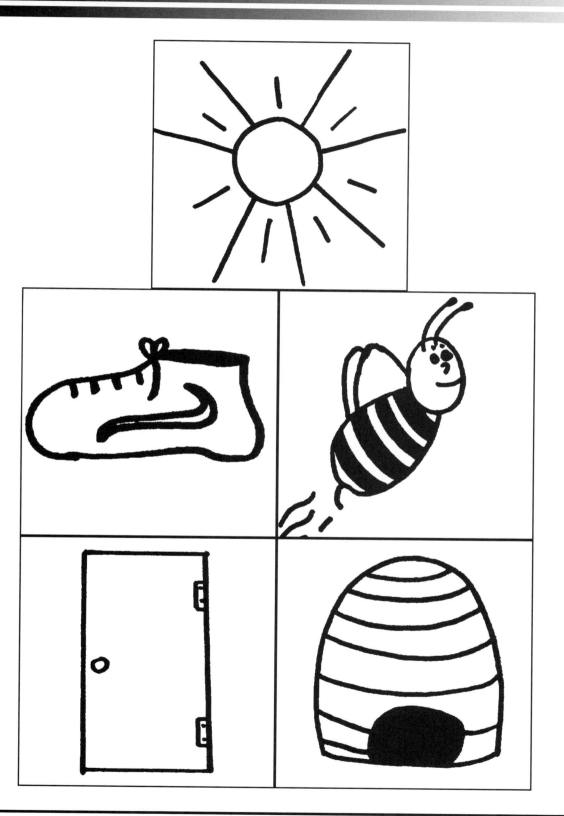

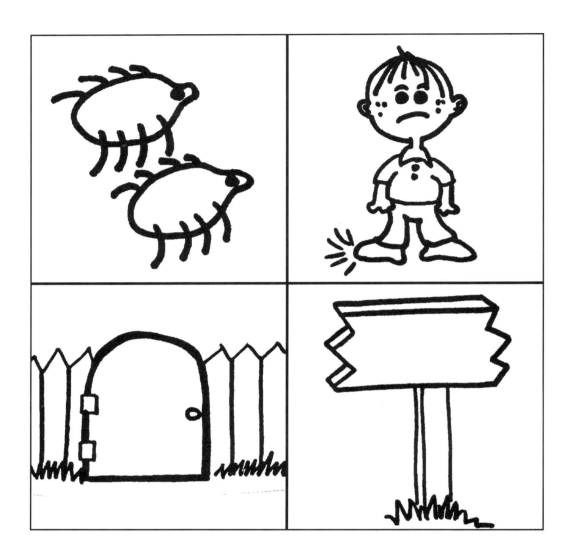

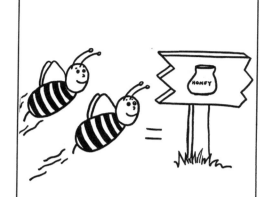

$$3 \times 3 = 9$$

(bee bee sign)
Two bees flying in a line,
Ahead they see a honey sign.
Three times three equals nine. 9.

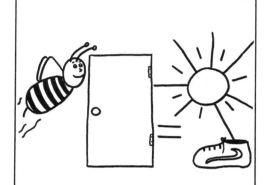

$$3 \times 4 = 12$$

(bee door sun shoe)
The bee by the door has a good view;
He sees the sun wearing the shoe.
Three times four is a one and a two. 12.

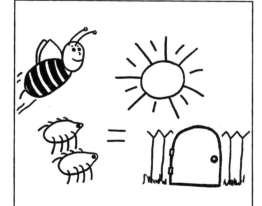

$$3 \times 6 = 18$$

(bee ticks sun gate)
The bee and ticks will not be late.
They hurry to sit in the sun by the gate.
Three times six is a one and an eight. 18.

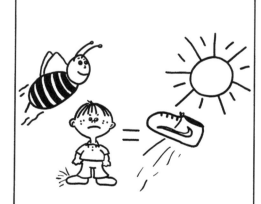

$$3 \times 7 = 21$$

(bee Kevin shoe sun)
The bee stung Kevin and that's no fun.
He's so mad he kicks his shoe at the sun.
Three times seven is a two and a one. 21.

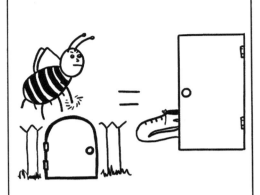

$$3 \times 8 = 24$$

(bee gate shoe door)
The bee by the gate has a foot that's sore.
He got his new shoe stuck in the door.
Three times eight is a two and a four. 24.

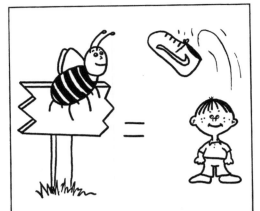

$$3 \times 9 = 27$$

(bee sign shoe Kevin)
The bee on the sign looks up toward heaven.
He sees the shoe fall that was kicked by Kevin.
Three times nine is a two and a seven. 27.

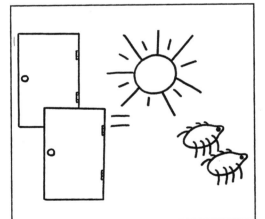

$$4 \times 4 = 16$$

(door door sun ticks)
Past the doors both made of sticks,
We see sun shining on the ticks.
Four times four is a one and a six. 16.

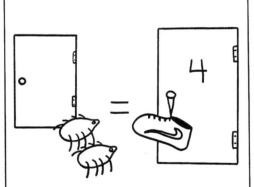

$$4 \times 6 = 24$$

(door ticks shoe door)
The ticks go past the little door
And hang a shoe on the door with the four.
Four times six is a two and a four. 24.

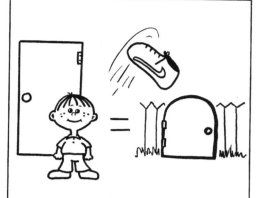

4 x 7 = 28

(door Kevin shoe gate)
Out of the door runs Kevin, late;
He kicks his shoe right at the gate.
Four times seven is a two and an eight. 28.

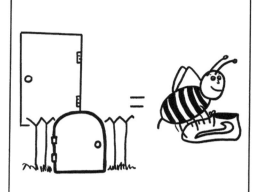

4 x 8 = 32

(door gate bee shoe)
Past one door and one gate, too,
We see the bee upon the shoe.
Four times eight is a three and a two. 32.

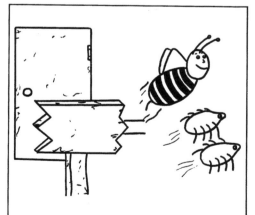

4 x 9 = 36

(door sign bee ticks)
The door and sign both have some nicks,
But not the little bee or ticks.
Four times nine is a three and a six. 36.

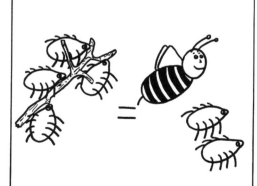

6 x 6 = 36

(ticks ticks bee ticks)
Ticks and ticks may nibble sticks,
But no sticks for this bee and ticks.
Six times six is a three and a six. 36.

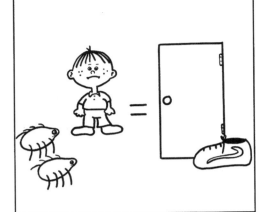

$$6 \times 7 = 42$$

(ticks Kevin door shoe)
Ticks and Kevin feeling blue,
See the door beside the shoe.
Six times seven is a four and a two. 42.

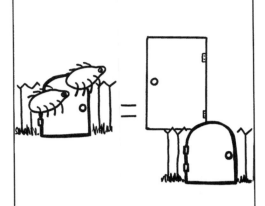

$$6 \times 8 = 48$$

(ticks gate door gate)
Ticks on the gate just sit and wait;
They cannot open a door or gate.
Six times eight is a four and an eight. 48.

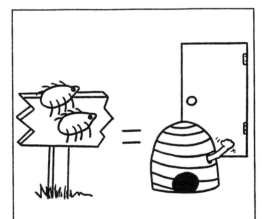

$$6 \times 9 = 54$$

(ticks sign hive door)
Ticks on a sign would surely roar
To see a hive knock on a door.
Six times nine is a five and a four. 54.

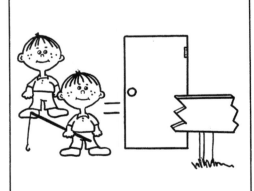

$$7 \times 7 = 49$$

(Kevin Kevin door sign)
Kevin and Kevin hold a fishing line,
While past the door they see a sign.
Seven times seven is a four and a nine. 49.

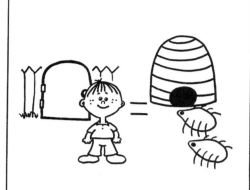

$7 \times 8 = 56$

(Kevin gate hive ticks)
Kevin stands by the gate doing tricks.
Watching him from the hive are the ticks.
Seven times eight is a five and a six. 56.

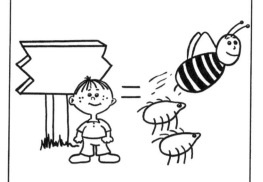

$7 \times 9 = 63$

(Kevin sign ticks bee)
Kevin goes past the sign to see
The little ticks beside the bee.
Seven times nine is a six and a three. 63.

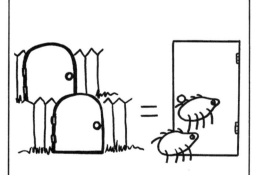

$8 \times 8 = 64$

(gate gate ticks door)
Past one gate then one gate more,
See the ticks rest on the door.
Eight times eight is a six and a four. 64.

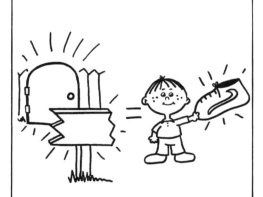

$8 \times 9 = 72$

(gate sign Kevin shoe)
The gate with the sign is bright and new,
And Kevin holds up his new shoe too.
Eight times nine is a seven and a two. 72.

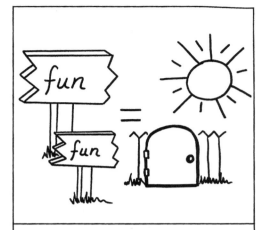

9 x 9 = 81

(sign sign gate sun)
Big sign and little sign both say fun.
It's fun to swing on a gate in the sun.
Nine times nine is an eight and a one. 81.

The author wishes to thank the following people who
contributed to this project:

Matthew Acosta, picture of air writing (pgs. 164 and 220), cop & dinosaur (pgs. 240-241), Figures 8a and 8b (pgs. 118, 119, 126, 131)

Simone Acosta & Judith Fuhrman, MFM pictures (pgs. 291-298)

John Benbow, hand grip pictures (p. 90) from *Hand Function and the Child*, ed. Henderson & Pehoski.

Judy Burkhart, airplane pictures (p. 244)

Josie Burns, song, *The Select Few*, (p. 18)

Travis Chung, 13 Colonies Rap (p. 287)

Richard Lederer, Tom Swifty, Croaker & reduplication games (pgs. 247-249)

Deedra Love-Dobis, visualization picture (p. 266)

Judy Love, MFM poems (pgs. 293-298), TREAT strategy (pgs. 187-190), subject/verb agreement activity (pgs. 243-245)

Martha S. Reed, Center for Development & Learning, University of North Carolina, Chapel Hill, for ideas on writing formats & suggestions for charts (Chapter 13)

RET Center Press, use of MFR pictures (pg. 159)

RET Center Press, use of information from *The Writing Dilemma*

Eli Richards for use of his story and work samples

Sally Smith, SAGE strategy (pgs. 204-207) and state unit (pgs. 249-250)

Colonel Stoopnagle, *Pea Little Thrigs* (pgs. 147 and 153-154)

Bibliography

Adams, J.J. *Beginning to Read: Thinking and Learning About Print*. Cambridge, MA: MIT Press, 1990.

Adams, Marilyn J., Lundberg, Ingvar, & Beeler, Terri. *Phonemic Awareness in Young Children*. Baltimore, MD: Paul H. Brookes, 1998.

Adams, Scott. Macworld Online: Chat with Scott Adams. *Dilbert™ Unbound*. 1996.

Bakker, D.J., Bouma, A., & Gardien, C.J. "Hemisphere-specific treatment of dyslexia subtypes: A field experiment." *Journal of Learning Disabilities*, 23, 1990:433-438.

Bear, Donald R. et al. *Words Their Way: Word Study for Phonics, Vocabulary, and Spelling*. Upper Saddle River, NJ: Prentice-Hall, 1996.

Behan, W.M., Behan, P.O., and Geschwind, N. "Anti-Rho Antibody in Mothers of Dyslexic Children." *Dev. Med. Child Neurology* 27, 1985:538-542.

Bell, Nanci & Lindamood, Phyllis. *Vanilla Vocabulary: A Visualized / Verbalized Vocabulary Book*. Paso Robles, CA: Academy of Reading Publications, 1993.

Bell, Nanci. *Visualizing and Verbalizing for Language Comprehension and Thinking*. Paso Robles, CA: Academy of Reading Publications, 1991.

Bissell, Julie, Fisher, Jean, Owens, Carol, & Polcyn, Patricia. *Sensory Motor Handbook: A Guide for Implementing and Modifying Activities in the Classroom*. Torrance, CA: Sensory Integration International, 1988.

Burgess, Thornton W. *Mother West Wind's Children*. Boston, MA: Little & Brown, 1985.

Butler, K.G. *Preschool Language Processing Performance and Later Reading Achievement* in Maslin, R.L. and Maslin, M.W. *Preschool Prevention of Reading Failure*. Timonium, MD: York Press, 1988.

California State Department of Education. *Teaching Reading: A Balanced, Comprehensive Approach to Teaching Reading in Prekindergarten Through Grade Three*. Sacramento, CA: California Department of Education, 1996.

Chase, Christopher H., Rosen, Glenn D., & Sherman, Gordon F. *Developmental Dyslexia: Neural, Cognitive & Genetic Mechanisms*. Baltimore, MD: York Press, 1996.

Churchill, W. *My Early Life* 1930, in West, 1997.

Clark, Diana Brewster, & Uhry, Joanna Kellogg. *Dyslexia: Theory and Practice of Remedial Instruction*, 2nd Ed. Baltimore, MD: York Press, 1995.

Clarke, Louise. *How to Recognize and Overcome Dyslexia in Your Child: Can't Read, Can't Write, Can't Talk Too Good Either*. New York: Penguin Books, 1973.

Cramer, Shirley C. & Ellis, William. *Learning Disabilities: Lifelong Issues*. Baltimore, MD: Paul H. Brookes Publishing Company, 1996.

Curriculum and Instruction Steering Committee. *Guide to the CA Reading Initiative*. Sacramento, CA: California County Superintendent Educ. Services Assoc., 1996.

Deshler, D. et al. *Teaching Adolescents with Learning Strategies and Methods*. Denver, CO: Love Publishing, 1996.

Deuel, R.K. "Developmental Dysgraphia and Motor Skill Disorders." *Journal of Child Neurology*. 10, 1994: 6-8.

Diamond, Linda & Mandel, Sheila. *Building a Powerful Reading Program: From Research to Practice*. Sacramento, CA: CSU Institute for Education Reform, 1996.

Ehri, L.C. "Grapheme-Phoneme Knowledge is Essential for Learning to Read Words in English." Dr. J. Metsala and L. Ehri (Eds.), *Word Recognition in Beginning Reading* (pp. 3-40). Hillsdale, NJ: Erlbaum, 1998.

Ellison, Launa. *The Brain: A User's Guide*. Tucson, AZ: Zephyr Press, 1995.

Fawcett, A.J., Singleton, C.H., & Peer, L. *Advances in Early Years: Screening for Dyslexia in the United Kingdom*. Annals of Dyslexia, Vol. 48. Baltimore, MD: International Dyslexia Association, 1998, pp. 57-88.

Fletcher, J.M., Francis, D.J., Rourke, B.P., Shaywitz, S.E., and Shaywitz, B.A. *Classification of Learning Disabilities: Relationships with Other Childhood Disorders*. In G.R. Lyon, D.B. Gray, J.F. Kavanagh, and N.A. Krasnegor (Eds.). *Better Understanding Learning Disabilities: New Views from Research and Their Implications for Education and Public Policies*. Baltimore, MD: Paul H. Brookes Publishing Co., 1993.

Foorman, B.R., Francis, D.J., Fletcher, J.M., Schatschneider, C., & Mehta, P. "The Role of Instruction in Learning to Read: Preventing Reading Failure in At-risk Children." *Journal of Educational Psychology*, Mar 90(1)1998:37-55

Francis, D.J., Fletcher, J.M., Rourke, B.P., Shaywitz, S.E., & Shaywitz, B.A. Cognitive profiles of reading disability: Comparisons of discrepancy and low achievement definitions. *Journal of Educational Psychology, 86*. 1994:6-23.

Gababurda, Albert M. *Dyslexia and Development: Neurobiological Aspects of Extra-Ordinary Brains*. Cambridge, MA: Harvard University Press, 1993.

Geschwind, Norman. "Orton Was Right." Maryland: International Dyslexia Association, 1982.

Gillingham, Anna, & Stillman, Bessie. *Remedial Training for Children with Specific Disability in Reading, Spelling, and Penmanship*. Cambridge, MA: Educators Publishing Service, Inc., revised 1998.

Gillingham, Anna, & Stillman, Bessie. *Remedial Training for Children with Specific Disability in Reading, Spelling, and Penmanship*. Cambridge, MA: Educators Publishing Service, Inc., 1968.

Bibliography

Greene, Ed.D., Jane Fell & Moats, Ed.E., Louisa Cook. *Testing: Critical Components in the Clinical Identification of Dyslexia.* International Dyslexia Association Emeritus Series. Baltimore, MD: International Dyslexia Association, 1995.

Greene, Victoria E. & Enfield, Ph.D., Mary Lee. *Project Read.* Bloomington, MN: Language Circle Enterprises, 1994.

Guarino, Deborah. *Is Your Mama a Llama?* New York: Scholastic, Inc., 1989.

Gupta, Kapil. *Human Brain Coloring Workbook: An Interactive Approach to Learning.* New York, NY: Princeton Review Publishing, 1997.

Haldy, M.S., OTR, Mary; & Haack, M.S., OTR, Laurel. *Making It Easy: Sensorimotor Activities at Home and School.* San Antonio, TX: Therapy Skill Builders, 1995.

Hall, Susan, and Moats, Ed.E., Louisa Cook. *Straight Talk About Reading: How Parents Can Make a Difference During the Early Years.* Chicago, IL: Contemporary Books, 1999.

Healy, Jane M. *Your Child's Growing Mind: A Guide to Brain Development and Learning from Birth to Adolescence.* NY: Bantam Books, 1987.

Henry, Marcia K. & Redding, Nancy C. *Patterns for Success in Reading and Spelling: A Multisensory Approach to Teaching Phonics and Word Analysis.* Austin, TX: Pro-Ed, 1995.

Hirsch, E.D., Kett, Joseph, Trefil, James. *The Dictionary of Cultural Literacy.* Boston, MA: Houghton Mifflin, 1988.

Holmes, Emily in Lally, Kath & Price, Debbie M. "The Brain Reads Sound by Sound." *The Sun*, Baltimore, MD: November 3, 1997.

IMSLEC (International Multisensory Structured Language Education Council). *Clinical Studies of Multisensory Structured Language Education for Students with Dyslexia and Related Disorders.* Salem, OR: IMSLEC, 1995.

International Dyslexia Association (IDA). *Perspectives*, 24:4, 1998:4.

Juel, Connie. *Learning to Read and Write in One Elementary School.* NY: Springer-Verlag, 1994.

Kemper, David, Nathan, Ruth, & Sebranek, Patrick. *Writer's Express.* Wilmington, MA: Great Source Educ. Co., 1995.

Kemper, David, Nathan, Ruth, & Sebranek, Patrick. *Write Away.* Wilmington, MA: Great Source Educ. Co., 1996.

Knight, M.S.Ed., Janice Miller; & Decker, B.S., OTR/L, Mary Jo Gilpin. *Hands at Work and Play: Developing Fine Motor Skills at School and Home.* San Antonio, TX: Therapy Skill Builders, 1994.

Lederer, Richard & Dowis, Richard. *The Write Way: The S.P.E.L.L. Guide to Real-Life Writing.* New York, NY: Pocket Books, 1995.

Lederer, Richard. *The Play of Words: Fun & Games for Language Lovers.* New York, NY: Pocket Books, 1990.

Lederer, Richard. *Get Thee to a Punnery.* Charleston, SC: Wyrick & Company, 1988.

Levine, Melvin D. "Bridges." Keynote Address at Learning Disability Association State Conference in San Francisco, CA, 1993.

Levine, Melvin D. *Developmental Variation and Learning Disorders.* Cambridge, MA: Educators Publishing Service, 1987.

Levine, Melvin D. *Developmental Variation and Learning Disorders,* 2nd ed. Cambridge, MA: Educators Publishing Service, 1998.

Liberman, I.Y., Shankweiler, D. "Phonology and beginning reading: A tutorial." In L. Rieben and C.A. Perfetti (Eds.), *Learning to Read: Basic Research and its Implications.* Hillsdale, NY: Lawrence Erlbaum Assoc., 1991.

Lindamood, Patricia C. & Phyllis D., *The Lindamood Phoneme Sequencing Program for Reading, Spelling, and Speech (LiPS).* Austin, TX: Pro-Ed, 1998.

Lyon, G. Reid. *Frames of Reference for the Assessment of Learning Disabilities: New Views on Measurement Issues.* Baltimore, MD: Paul H. Brookes Publishing Co., 1994.

Lyon, G. Reid. "Recent Discoveries in Reading Disabilities." Speech at International Orton Dyslexia Society Conference, Houston, TX, 1995.

Lyon, G. Reid. "Toward a Definition of Dyslexia." *Annals of Dyslexia* 45 1995:3-26.

Lyon, G. Reid. "Research initiatives in learning disabilities: Contributions from scientists supported by the National Institute of Child Health and Human Development." *Journal of Child Neurology* 10, 1995:120-126.

Lyon, G. Reid. "The State of Research" in Cramer, S.C. and Ellis, W., *Learning Disabilities: Lifelong Issues.* Baltimore, MD: Paul H. Brookes, 1996.

Lyon, G. Reid. *Learning to Read: A Call from Research to Action.* Their World 1997/1998. New York, NY: National Center for Learning Disabilities, 1997, pp. 16-25.

Maccarone, Grace. *What is That? Said the Cat.* New York: Scholastic, Inc., 1995.

Margulies, Nancy. *Mapping Inner Space: Learning and Teaching Mind Mapping.* Tucson, AZ: Zephyr Press, 1991.

Martin, Jr., Bill. *When It Rains, It Rains.* New York: Holt, Rinehart, Winston, 1970.

Moats, Louisa Cook. *Spelling: Development, Disability, and Instruction.* MD: York Press, 1995.

Moats, Louisa C. "Teaching decoding." *American Educator*, Summer 1998.

Orton-Gillingham—See Gillingham

Bibliography

Pehrsson, Robert S. & Robinson, H. Alan. *Semantic Organizers: A Study Strategy for Special Needs Learners.* Rockville, MD: Aspen Publication, 1985.

Pehrsson, Robert S. & Robinson, H. Alan. *The Semantic Organizer Approach to Writing and Reading Instruction.* Rockville, MD: Aspen Publication, 1985.

Pehrsson, Robert S. & Robinson, H. Alan. *The Semantic Organizer.* Rockville, MD: Aspen Publication, 1989.

Pennington, B.F. *Diagnosing Learning Disorders: A Neurological Framework.* New York: Guilford Press, 1991.

Pollack, Cecelia and Branden, Ann. "Odyssey of a 'Mirrored' Personality." An Interdisciplinary Journal of the Orton Dyslexia Society. *Annals of Dyslexia,* Vol. XXXII 1982:282.

Rawson, Margaret B. *Dyslexia Over the Lifespan: A 55-year longitudinal study.* Cambridge, MA: Educators Publishing Service, Inc., 1995.

Reading Program Advisory. *Teaching Reading: A Balanced, Comprehensive Approach to Teaching Reading in Pre-Kindergarten Through Grade Three.* Sacramento, CA: CA Dept. of Education Publishing, 1996.

Reed, Martha. Handout from Learning Disability Workshop at the University of North Carolina at Chapel Hill, 1995.

RET Dyslexia Diagnostic System. Riverside, CA: RET Center Press, 1998.

Richards, Regina. *LEARN: Playful Techniques to Accelerate Learning.* Tucson, AZ: Zephyr Press, 1993 (out of print).

Richards, Regina. *Memory Foundations for Reading: A visual mnemonic system for sound/symbol correspondence.* Riverside, CA: RET Center Press, 1997.

Robertson, Carolyn & Salter, Wanda. *The Phonological Awareness Test.* LinguiSystems, Inc., 1995.

Rockefeller, Nelson. Quote in *TV Guide.* Oct. 16, 1976.

Rose, Laura. *Picture This: Teaching Reading Through Visualization.* Tucson, AZ: Zephyr Press, 1989.

Rose, Laura. *Picture This for Beginning Readers: Teaching Reading Through Visualization.* Tucson, AZ: Zephyr Press, 1991.

Rubin, Bonnie Miller. *Chicago Tribune* 3/2/97 "Reading Wars," quoting G. Reid Lyon, Ph.D., Director, NICHD.

Schumaker, J.B., Nolan, S.B., & Deshler, D.D. *Error Monitoring Strategies: Instructor's Manual.* Lawrence, KS: University of Kansas Institute for Research in Learning Disabilities, 1985.

Sedita, Joan. *Landmark Study Skills Guide.* Prides Crossing, MA: Landmark Foundation, 1989.

Share, D. & Stanovich, K. "Cognitive Processes in Early Reading Development: Accommodating Individual Differences into a Mode of Acquisition," *Issues in Education:* Contributions from *Educational Psychology*, Vol. 1 (1995), pp. 1-57.

Shaywitz, B.A., Fletcher, J.M., Holahan, J.M., & Shaywitz, S.E. Discrepancy compared to low achievement definitions of reading disability: Results of the Connecticut longitudinal study. *Journal of Learning Disabilities.* 1992: 25, 639-648.

Silverstein, Shel. *A Light in the Attic.* New York: Harper & Row, 1981.

Silverstein, Shel. *Falling Up.* New York: Harper Collins Publ., 1996.

Simon, Seymour. *The Brain: Our Nervous System.* New York: Morrow Junior Books, 1997.

Simpson, Eileen. *Reversals: A Personal Account of Victory Over Dyslexia.* Boston: Houghton Mifflin Co., 1979.

Slingerland, Beth H. *A Multisensory Approach to Language Arts for Specific Language Disability Children: A Guide for Primary Teachers.* Cambridge, MA: Educators Publishing Service, Inc., 1977.

Smith, B.K. *The Dilemma of a Dyslexic Man.* Hogue Foundation for Mental Health, The University of Texas at Austin, 1968.

Stanovich, Keith E. Toward an interactive-compensatory model of individual differences in the development of reading fluency. *Reading Research Quarterly.* 1980: 16,32-71.

Stanovich, K.E. "The Right and Wrong Places to Look for the Cognitive Locus of Reading Disability." *Annals of Dyslexia*, Vol. 38 1998: 154-180.

Stanovich, Keith E. "Romance and Reality," *The Reading Teacher.* 47:4, December 1993/January 1994.

Stanovich, K.E. "Cognitive Science Meets Beginning Reading." *Psychological Science,* 2, 1991: 70-81.

Talan, Jamie. *Newsday*, July 29, 1998:A24.

Tarricone, Jean Gudaitis. *The Landmark Method for Teaching Writing.* Prides Crossing, MA: Landmark Foundation, 1995.

Texas Scottish Rite Hospital for Children. *Dyslexia Training Program.* Dallas Texas Child Development Department, 1993.

The Pencil Grip. Los Angeles, CA: All the Write News.

Thomasson, Melissa. Address at 1993 Dimensions of Dyslexia Conference, Southern California Consortium of The Orton Dyslexia Society, 1993.

Torgesen, J.K. *The Learning Disabled Child as an Inactive Learner: Topics in Learning and Learning Disabilities*, 2:455, 1982.

Bibliography

Torgesen, Joseph K. & Bryan, Brian R. *Phonological Awareness Training for Reading*. Austin, TX: Pro-Ed, 1994.

Torgesen, Joseph K. Catch them before they fall. *American Educator*, Summer 1998.

Torgesen, Joseph K. "The New Research on Reading: Implications for Practice." Presentation at *Dimensions of Dyslexia*, Southern California Consortium, International Dyslexia Association Conference, April 17, 1999.

Vellutino, Frank R. & Scanlon, Donna M. *Diagnosing Reading Disability Through Early Intervention*. Their World 1997/1998. New York, NY: National Center for Learning Disabilities, 1997, pp. 36-38.

Wallach, G.P. & Butler, K.G. (Eds.). *Language Learning Disabilities in School Age Children*. New York: Williams and Wilkins, 1984.

West, Thomas G. *In the Mind's Eye: Visual Thinkers, Gifted People with Dyslexia and Other Learning Difficulties, Computer Images and the Ironies of Creativity*. New York: Prometheus Books, 1997.

Yopp, Hallie Kay. *Developing Phonemic Awareness in Young Children*. The Reading Teacher 45:9, May 1992. 696-703.

Index

23-07-12